Psychology and Sociology
for GNM and BPT Students

Other books by the author under JAYPEE banner:

1. Psychology for Graduate Nurses
2. Biochemistry for Nurses
3. Nutrition and Biochemistry for Nurses
4. Sociology for Graduate Nurses
5. Microbiology for Graduate Nurses
6. Practical Record Book for GNM

Psychology and Sociology
for GNM and BPT Students

Third Edition

Jacob Anthikad
MA (Psy) BEd MA (Chem) DTech (Biochem)

Retired Wing Commander
Indian Air Force (IAF)
Bengaluru, Karnataka, India

Visiting Professor
Kempegowda College of Nursing
MS Ramaiah College of Nursing
St. John's College of Nursing
St. Philomena's College of Nursing
Bengaluru, Karnataka, India

JAYPEE

JAYPEE BROTHERS MEDICAL PUBLISHERS
The Health Sciences Publisher
New Delhi | London

Jaypee Brothers Medical Publishers (P) Ltd

Headquarters

Jaypee Brothers Medical Publishers (P) Ltd
4838/24, Ansari Road, Daryaganj
New Delhi 110 002, India
Phone: +91-11-43574357
Fax: +91-11-43574314
Email: jaypee@jaypeebrothers.com

Overseas Offices

J.P. Medical Ltd
83 Victoria Street, London
SW1H 0HW (UK)
Phone: +44-2031708910
Fax: +02-03-0086180
Email: info@jpmedpub.com

Jaypee Medical Inc
The Bourse
111 South Independence Mall East
Suite 835, Philadelphia, PA 19106, USA
Phone: + 267-519-9789
Email: joe.rusko@jaypeebrothers.com

Jaypee Brothers Medical Publishers (P) Ltd
Shorakhute, Kathmandu, Nepal
Phone: +00977-9841528578
Email: jaypee.nepal@gmail.com

Jaypee-Highlights Medical Publishers Inc
City of Knowledge, Bld. 237, Clayton
Panama City, Panama
Phone: +507-301-0496
Fax: +507-301-0499
Email: cservice@jphmedical.com

Jaypee Brothers Medical Publishers (P) Ltd
17/1-B Babar Road, Block-B, Shaymali
Mohammadpur, Dhaka-1207
Bangladesh
Mobile: +08801912003485
Email: jaypeedhaka@gmail.com

Website: www.jaypeebrothers.com
Website: www.jaypeedigital.com

Inquiries for bulk sales may be solicited at: jaypee@jaypeebrothers.com

Psychology and Sociology for GNM and BPT Students

First Edition: 2006
Second Edition: 2009
Third Edition: 2014
Reprint: **2024**

ISBN 978-93-5090-984-3

Printed at: Sterling Graphics Pvt. Ltd.

Dedicated to

My brother the Rev Nicholas Anthikad

MA (Novo Scotia) MSc (Chennai) STL (Rome)

Former Principal

St Thomas College

Thrissur, Kerala, India

PREFACE TO THE THIRD EDITION

The different data included in the second edition have been updated as per the figures of Census 2011–12. The question bank has also been completed by including the Board Question Papers for the period February 2009 to June 2013 to make this popular textbook more useful for the students and nursing faculty. Suggestions from the users are most welcome and will be included in the subsequent editions.

The author is grateful to Shri Jitendar P Vij (Group Chairman), Mr Ankit Vij (Managing Director) and Mr Tarun Duneja (Director-Publishing) of M/s Jaypee Brothers Medical Publishers (P) Ltd, New Delhi, India, and Mr V Venugopal (Branch Manager, Bengaluru), for their encouragement and constant support.

Jacob Anthikad
Wing Commander (Retd)

PREFACE TO THE FIRST EDITION

The Indian Nursing Council, in their latest syllabus, introduced a separate paper for Behavioural Sciences in II GNM, recognising the growing relevance of psychology and sociology in the field of nursing. This book is an honest attempt to have a combined volume to meet the requirements of students and teachers for the GNM course as well as Bachelor of Physiotherapy. I hope that this latest book of mine will receive the same enthusiastic welcome like my earlier works.

Words cannot express my sincere sense of gratitude to Shri Jitendar P Vij (Chairman and Managing Director) of M/s Jaypee Brothers Medical Publishers (P) Ltd, New Delhi, India, Mr Tarun Duneja (General Manager-Publishing) and Mr RN Mandal (Regional Manager), Bengaluru, who encouraged me to author this book.

Suggestions and criticisms are always welcome and will be incorporated in future revised edition.

Jacob Anthikad
Wing Commander (Retd)

CONTENTS

PART I: PSYCHOLOGY

PART II: SOCIOLOGY

INDIAN NURSING COUNCIL SYLLABUS 2001

PAPER II: BEHAVIOURAL SCIENCES

PSYCHOLOGY

Time: 40 Hours

Course Description

This course is designed to help students understand the dynamics of human behaviour and concept of mental health. This will enable them to develop positive attitude and good interpersonal relationships in the practice of nursing in all health care settings.

General Objectives

Upon completion of this course, the students will be able to:

- Describe the concept of mental health and psychology
- Explain the dynamics of human behaviour, personality and learning
- Discuss the role of adjustment mechanisms and emotions in health and illness
- Demonstrate skills in the application of principle of psychology in nursing practice in all kinds of health care settings.

Course Contents

Unit I: Introduction

Definition, scope of psychology and its importance in nursing profession.

Unit II: Psychology of Human Behaviour

- Dynamics of behaviour, motivation and behavioural process of adjustment, adjustments and maladjustments, unconscious behaviour

- Frustration: Sources and nature of frustration, measures to overcome frustration
- Conflicts: Types, unconscious conflict, resolution, conflict and nursing
- Adjustment mechanism: Meaning, types and importance
- Emotions: In health and disease, emotional situations, control of emotions, effect of emotional reactions on health
- Attitudes: Meaning, development, changes in attitude, attitude and nursing
- Habits: Formation, types, effective habit formation, advantages and disadvantages of habit formation.

Unit III: Learning

- Nature of learning, laws and types of learning, factors promoting effective learning, memory and forgetfulness
- Thinking and reasoning
- Nature and type of thinking
- Problem solving and reasoning.

Unit IV: Observation

Attention and perception, factors affection attention and observation and errors in perception.

Unit V: Intelligence

- Definition, individual differences in intelligence
- Mental ability and nature of intelligence
- Measurement of intelligence
- Development of intelligence behaviour.

Unit VI: Personality

- Meaning, types, factors affecting development of personality
- Characteristics of various age group: Child, adolescent, adult and aged
- Will and character

SOCIOLOGY

Time: 20 Hours

Course Description

This course is designed to help student gain an understanding of sociology in the context of its relevance to nursing practice.

General Objectives

Upon completion of this course, the students will be able to:
- Describe the concept of the family as a social unit and the status of the individual in the family
- Explain the dynamics of society and identify common social problems
- Demonstrate ability to understand the sociocultural and economic aspects of the community in the light of their effects on health and illness
- Utilise the knowledge and understanding of sociology in nursing practice.

Course Contents

Unit I: Introduction

- Concept, scope nature and importance of sociology in nursing.
- The sociocultural and economic aspects of the community and their effects in health and illness.

Unit II: The Individual

- Brief review of human growth and development
- Effect of environment on childhood, adolescence, adulthood and old age
- The right and responsibilities of the individual in a democratic society.

Unit III: The Family

- Family as a social institution and basic unit for health services
- Basic needs of family, its structure and relationships
- Family life education: Premarriage, marriage and parenthood.

Unit IV: The Society

- Concept
- Group: Types, structure, inter-group relationship, group cycle, group behaviour and group morale
- Social changes, social control, social stratification
- Rural and urban society
- Social problems: Unmarried mothers, dowry system, prostitution, drug addiction, alcoholism, delinquency, handicapped, child abuse, women abuse
- Social agencies and remedial measures.

Unit V: The Community

Definition, characteristics and culture.

Unit VI: Economy

- Resources of the country: Natural, occupational, agricultural, industrial, etc.
- Social security
- Population explosion: Its effect on economy and the need for population control
- Budgeting for a family, per capita income and its impact on health and illness.

PART—I

PSYCHOLOGY

1. Definition, Methods and Scope: Psychology and Nursing
2. Behaviour and Its Dynamics: Behavioural Process of Adjustment
3. Motivation: The "Why" of Behaviour
4. Frustration and Conflicts
5. Defence Mechanisms or Adjustment Mechanisms
6. Emotions in Health and Disease
7. Attitudes: The Way We See Things
8. Habits and Skills
9. The Learning Process
10. Remembering and Forgetting
11. Thinking and Reasoning
12. Observation: Attention, Sensation and Perception
13. Intelligence and Its Measurement
14. Personality and Its Development
15. Developing Personality: Different Age Groups
16. Will and Character

1 Definition, Methods and Scope: Psychology and Nursing

INTRODUCTION

The beginnings of psychology are to be found in the curiosity of primitive man about himself and his companions. The development of psychology as a science has followed a long and somewhat uncertain course through the centuries. The early Greek philosophers like Aristotle (384–322 BC) and Hippocrates (460–370 BC) (Father of medicine) made many contributions.

DEFINITION OF PSYCHOLOGY

It was in the year 1590 that Rudolf Geockle used the word Psychology. It is derived from two Greek words "*Psyche*" and "*Logos*". "*Psyche*" means soul or spirit. "*Logos*" means knowledge or study of. Psychology thus was the study of the soul. The word soul was used vaguely and attained religious significance with the rise of Christianity. Therefore, William James (1842-1910) used the term "mind" in place of soul in 1890. But this definition also became unsatisfactory because mind was abstract and could not be seen or understood, unless what the mind did was seen. Behaviour is what the mind does. Therefore, psychology is defined as the scientific study of behaviour and mental processes.

Defining psychology as the scientific study of behaviour does not exclude mind and other internal processes from the field of psychology; what a person does—his or her behaviour—is the outcome of the internal mental processes.

Psychology is a Positive Science

A science is a body of systematized knowledge that is gathered carefully observing and measuring events. Psychologists do experiments and make observations which others can repeat and verify. It is this method of science that distinguishes psychology from art and philosophy. Objectivity, reliability, validity and predictability are characteristics of science.

Behaviour includes all human activities—motor activities like walking and speaking, cognitive activities such as perceiving, remembering, thinking or reasoning and emotional activities like feeling happy, angry or sad. Behaviour includes all our reactions and responses to the environmental stimuli. Behaviour is anything that can be observed.

Psychology is related to many other behavioural sciences like anthropology (study of man in different cultures), sociology (study of human behaviour in a group) geography, history and economics which study various aspects of human behaviour.

Psychology is a very young science having separated from philosophy in 1879 when Wilhelm Wundt (1832–1920) established the first psychological laboratory in the University of Leipzig, Germany. *Wundt was the first to measure human behaviour accurately and is called the "Father of Psychology"*. Thichener, James, Pavlov, Watson, Skinner, Freud, Rogers and Maslow were all important in the different areas of development of psychology as a science.

Methods of Psychology or Methods of Study of Behaviour

Introspection or Self-Observation Method

To introspect means to look within. It is internal perception or self observation. The individual himself observes his internal activities and processes whenever and wherever he likes to do so. It is indispensable for the study of internal behaviour. For example, a patient after an operation may be asked to report how he feels. The patient will try to look within and recall what happened and how he is feeling now.

Introspection does not involve any expenditure as it does not need any laboratory or apparatus. We get a direct knowledge of the mental experience of the individual. But the method cannot be used by children or mental defectives. It is highly subjective. It is a purely private affair and cannot be verified by other observers.

The Observation Method or Systematic Observation

It consists of collection of data by means of observing behaviour by somebody other than that person. For example, when a nurse is asked to make an observational report on a patient with an undiagnosed illness, she reports her observations such as the patient's temperature, pulse, colour, facial expression, restlessness, etc. Observation of the patient is very important in clinical medicine. The method is widely used also in studying the behaviour of children and animals.

The Experimental Method

In this method, made popular by Wundt, the psychologist studies, under controlled conditions, the effects of a dependent variable of changes in an independent variable. Many experiments are being conducted on people and animals dealing with learning, forgetting and many other mental activities. The tremendous progress of psychology during the twentieth century is mainly due to this method. For example, the famous Hawthorne experiment (1927-34) conducted in Western Electric Company, USA, by Elton Mayo, to find out in what circumstances production could be improved. Five girls participated. One by one factory conditions were altered, e.g. illumination, seating arrangements, rest pauses, etc.

The experimental method controls all variables. Examples are studying the effect of noise on learning, effect of a drug on sleep, etc. The following are the steps in an experiment:

1. Identifying a problem.
2. Formulation of the hypothesis.
3. Distinction between independent and dependent variables.
4. Arranging the environment and collection of data.
5. Analysis of the data.
6. Testing of the hypothesis by the result of the experiment.

The advantage of this method is that experiments can be repeated and results confirmed. It is highly objective. Limitations are that it cannot always be used, especially if the experiment might be dangerous to the subjects and are obtained in artificial situations. The method costs money and time and requires a laboratory.

The Survey Method or Inventory Method

This method uses questionnaires, checklists, rating scales, ranking and inventories to assess different aspects of behaviour, emotional experiences and aptitudes. It is also used for problems that cannot be directly observed. Surveys are used to gather information about political opinion, customer preferences, health needs and sexual behaviour. The results of a survey of a large number of people have to be carefully analysed before conclusions are made.

The Test Method

Abilities, interests, attitudes and intelligence are measured by this method by making use of carefully devised and standardised tests. The test can be administered to a large number of personnel at the same time saving a lot of time, energy and dislocation of routine work, e.g. intelligence tests, aptitude tests.

The Case History or Clinical Method

It is used regularly in the medical and nursing setting. It aims at studying the causes and basis of people's anxieties, fears and personal maladjustments. It makes use of case histories, interviews, home visits and psychological tests for that purpose. It gathers information about one patient, or a small group of patients from what the subject can recall, and also from all available sources like parents, sublings, teachers, schoolmates and school records and other written documents.

The Genetic or Developmental Method

It studies the growth of behaviour. For example, to understand the learning behaviour of an adult, the study will start from his childhood and adolescence.

Subfields of Psychology or Scope of Psychology

1. *Clinical psychology* is the largest subfield of psychology (55%). It is the study of techniques which are employed in the diagnosis and treatment of mentally and emotionally abnormal personalities. A clinical psychologist has a MA or PhD in psychology and is trained to apply psychotherapeutic techniques, to diagnose psychological disorders and to conduct tests and do research. However, being not a doctor, he cannot prescribe medicines. Psychiatrists are doctors holding a MD degree, specialised in behavioural problems. Being a physician, he uses drugs and other medical methods for treating the mentally ill. Psychoanalysis is different from clinical psychology and psychiatry. A psychoanalyst uses the special psychotherapeutic techniques developed by Sigmund Freud.
2. *Counselling psychology* is similar to clinical psychology but deals with people with relatively mild personal or emotional problems. Educational psychology deals with the learning problems and their remedies. Industrial and organisational psychology applies psychological principles to industry.
3. *Social psychology* deals with the behaviour of an individual as it is influenced by others and how an individual influences others' behaviour. It studies various types of group phenomena like public opinion, propaganda, attitudes, beliefs and crowd behaviour.
4. *Experimental psychology* involves basic research into the fundamental causes of human behaviour by studying such basic processes as learning and memory, sensation, perception, and motivation. Physiological psychology concerns the structure and functions of sense organs, nervous system, muscles and glands underlying all behaviour. It lays emphasis on the influence of bodily factors on human behaviour.
5. *Developmental psychology* studies the behaviour as it develops from birth, through childhood, adolescence and maturity to old age. It studies the factors that influence the growth or development of human behaviour. Child psychology studies the behaviour of children from birth to about age 12.

6. *Abnormal psychology* deals with the behaviour of individuals who are unusual. It studies mental disorders, their causes and treatment.
7. *Community psychology* is a broad field where social problems and the attempts of people to adapt to their work and community living are studied in the light of the principles of general psychology.

Psychology and the Student Nurse

Psychology has become an integral part of every profession including nursing. The study of human behaviour is of great value to a student nurse in a number of ways:

1. *It will help her understand herself*: She will get an insight into her motives, desires, emotions and ambitions. She will realise how her personality is highly individualistic and complex, how she arrives at decisions in her life and how she solves her problems. By knowing her strength and weaknesses, she can best use her own personality characteristics. This will let her direct her own life more productively and relate more easily with others, enabling her to control situations and attain self-discipline.
2. *It will help her to understand other people:* Leading to personal and professional adjustment. She will become sympathetic, alert, hardworking and love humanity. She will become emotionally mature, cultivate an active mind and habits and enjoy team work. The student nurse has to study, work and live with other nurses, doctors, patients and their families. With her scientific knowledge of human nature, she will understand them better and thus achieve greater success in interpersonal relationships.
3. *It will help her to improve situations by helping others solve their problems:* Illness and physical handicaps often bring about the need for major adjustments. Many diseases such as heart diseases and cancer are not cured by medical treatment, but are instead controlled. These diseases are for life and require special coping skills and health care. A nurse trained in educational psychology can be an effective health educator and can help in this kind of adjustments. In the

health care setting, the patient's role in treatment is a major factor. A good understanding of the patient by the nurse can be the best social support to patients who are hospitalised and also while coping with chronic mental illness.

4. An understanding of psychology can be of great help to a nurse to become a good health teacher to explain to the patient and relatives:
   a. The nature and diagnostic examination, findings and treatment.
   b. Principles of health and prevention of diseases.
   c. After care programmes and rehabilitation.
5. *She will understand the close relationship of body, mind and spirit*: She will recognise how her emotions affect her body and she will recognise the same in her patients. This will help her to control her life and recognise the similar needs in her patients.

QUESTIONS

1. How would you define psychology? What is its scope? Bring out its relationships with other sciences.
2. Explain the term "behaviour". What are the methods to study behaviour?
3. What is the nature and scope of psychology with reference to nursing?
4. Discuss in detail the case history of a patient you have studied. Give the psychological interpretation of his behaviour as observed by you.
5. Why is knowledge of psychology essential for a nurse?
6. With which professional in psychology would you seek help for the following:
   a. Serious mental illness (psychiatrist)
   b. Problem in relationship at work (Counsellor)
   c. Difficulty in adjusting to new sitation (Psychologist).

2 Behaviour and Its Dynamics: Behavioural Process of Adjustment

Human behaviour is the subject matter of psychology and is related to community health. Human behaviour is the interaction between physical and mental factors (body and mind). All forms of behaviour are responses to stimuli. Psychology attempts to study the relationship between stimuli and responses.

Stimuli

Stimuli are causes of our behaviour and are very varied and include:

a. *Environmental stimuli*: Like vision, touch and smell reach the cerebral cortex through nerve impulses. The information received is analysed and evaluated. By a set of another impulses the cerebral cortex "orders" the behaviour of the individual. The behaviour will be in conformation with the values, standards and expectations of the society. For example, nurse's behaviour towards her patients. A person's behaviour will be different under different situations.
b. *Emotions and feelings*: Behaviour is also dependent on our feelings and emotions. These stimuli arise within our body. When a person is blind with rage or paralysed by fear, he is a victim of his own emotions. Emotions thus affect our behaviour.
c. *Needs*: An individual's behaviour is also influenced by his needs, wants, desires or urges.
d. *Motivation*: Motivations are inner forces which drive an individual to a specific goal. Motives determine human behaviour.
e. *Intellectual perception*: A person's intellectual perceptions, thinking and reasoning can influence his behaviour in a given situation. Each individual behaves in ways which make sense to him.

Responses

The vaious responses to stimuli are classified as:

a. *Physical responses*: Such as habits and skills
b. *Organic responses*: Such as emotion, feelings, tension
c. *Intellectual responses*: Thinking, perception, reasoning.

ADJUSTMENT

Behaviour is also described as an adjustment to meet the needs of a given situation.

Adjustment is defined as the continuous process of satisfying one's desires, and it involves many aspects of behaviour. No one achieves a complete adjustment for a long period. Eventually, one need or the other arises and the individual must find ways of satisfying it.

Adjustment is a Process

Adjustment is a continuous process, not a fixed or static state. It exists on a continuum. At one end is the well adjusted person who is able to adapt as new needs arise. At the other end, is the poorly-adjusted person who may show signs of anxiety, aggression or disordered thinking. Usually, this person is less adaptive.

Adequate Adjustment

Sigmund Freud described mental health as expressing oneself in love and work. The well-adjusted person forms affectionate relationships and lives productively.

Erik Erikson considered adjustment as a lifelong process. Adjustment is the result of resolution of crisis at successive life stages.

Abraham Maslow described the well-adjusted person in terms of self-actualization. Human beings constantly seek expression of their full potential.

Carl Rogers identified two dimensions of the adjustment process, openness to experience and trust in ourself. Under these conditions human beings know to do what is appropriate at a given situation.

Characteristics of a Well-adjusted Person

1. He feels comfortable about himself
2. He feels right towards others
3. He is able to meet the demands of life
4. To meet the above standards he must possess:
   a. Awareness of himself
   b. Satisfying relationships with others
   c. Capacity for hard work
   d. Ability to give and take
   e. Knowledge of his strength and weaknesses
   f. Behaviour which is generally acceptable to others
   g. Respect for others
   h. Benefits of rest and sleep.

Personal and Professional Adjustment by Nurses

Any person who makes a living by doing something is a professional in that area of work. Professional nursing means that the person who requires training and higher education to practice the profession of nursing. The act of something fit to look right is called adjustment. As a person becomes a nurse, she becomes a member of a profession and will have to learn to adjust to the profession as well. This is what we call as professional adjustment.

Making Adjustments

Behaviour is an adjustment to meet the needs of a given situation. For examples, when a person does not succeed in something there are different ways he/she can react.

a. Losing temper and complaining to everyone
b. Avoiding others by isolating oneself
c. Making excuses for the failure

d. Accepting failure with grace and making amends by changing behaviour. Adjustment is both active and passive.

A successful nurse is one who is well adjusted and has the following qualities:

1. Likes people
2. Emotionally mature
3. Keen observation
4. Active mind and habits
5. Enjoys work.

Not everyone can make a good nurse. Only those who are sympathetic by nature, love humanity and are not afraid of hard work can become successful nurses making good adjustment to their profession. They are totally dedicated to the service of humanity and learn from their environment. Life of the nurse is very demanding. Constant advances in medicine, sociology, psychology and public health must keep her alert. She must do self-evaluation of her work and show the interest and will for improvement. She must extend these qualities for growth of her personal and professional life.

She may get very little time for herself. She must carefully plan to meet her recreational needs also.

Adjustments for Student Nurses

Following are some of the areas where student nurses will need early adjustment:

a. Living together in nurses' hostel-community life
b. Effectively deal with home sickness
c. Healthy personal habits
d. Social adjustment
e. Accepting responsibility
f. Punctuality
g. Principles of learning from textbooks, journals, obsevation, demonstrations and clinical exposures
h. Healthy study habits
i. How to take examination
j. Evaluation and counselling.

Forms of Maladjustments

Many disorders especially that of moderate severity can be considered from various perspectives. The various anxiety disorders include:

a. Generalized anxiety disorders in which there are no other specific symptoms except anxiety
b. Phobic disorders involving some incapacitating fear of an harmless object, and
c. Obsessive compulsive disorder (OCD) in which there are unwarranted but recurrent thoughts and/or action.

In many psychosomatic disorders, psychological stress has caused physical symptoms.

Unconscious Behaviour

Unconscious motivation refers to the influence of repressed thoughts, desires or impulses on our conscious thoughts and behaviours. Freud assumed that free association, dream interpretation and slip of the tongue reveal our unconscious. For example, if ten people witness an accident, we get 10 conflicting reports of the accident. This is because perceptions, prejudices and ideas which are unconscious and outside the control of those witnesses.

3 Motivation: The "Why" of Behaviour

Psychology deals with not only what people do but also, why they do so. Motivation literally means to move, to energise or to activate. Motivation is defined as 'conditions within the organism which arouse, maintain and direct behaviour towards a specific goal.' It is a driving or pulling force which results in persistent behaviour directed towards a particular goal. It is internal and is a vector quantity.

The word "motive" is commonly used to mean motivation. Generally, motivation is made up of motives or drives. Motives are expressions of a person's needs, hence they are personal and internal. Incentives are external. Motives are inferences from observations of behaviour. They are powerful tools for the explanation of behaviour, and they allow us to make predictions about future behaviour. Motives are the "dynamos" of human behaviour.

CLASSIFICATION OR TYPES OF MOTIVES

There are three kinds of motives—primary, stimulus and secondary or learned. Primary motives are called physiological or basic needs as they are necessary for survival of any organism—human, animal or plant. They are caused by the needs of our bodies. The main primary motives are hunger, thirst, avoidance of pain, need for air and sleep, elimination of wastes, regulation of body temperature and sex. All these are unlearned motives inborn in the organism.

Stimulus motives are also inborn but are not necessary for survival. They include activity, curiosity, exploration, manipulation and physical contact.

Primary Motives

Primary motives are essential for survival. They must be satisfied to some reasonale extent, before one can take up any other activity. Primary motives come to action when the physiological balance of the body is upset. This balance is called homeostasis.

Motives

Primary or biological or basic	Stimulus	Secondary, social or learned
Hunger	Activity	Achievement
Thirst	Curiosity	Affiliation
Avoidance of pain	Exploration	Aggression
Need for sleep and air	Manipulation	Power
Elimination of waste	Physical contact	Curiosity
Regulation of temperature		
Sex		

Hunger drive: When the food supply of the body is exhausted, certain biochemical changes take place in the tissues of the body. This causes the stomach to contract which gives hunger pains. The hunger must be satisfied in order to help the body to return to a physiological balance or homeostasis.

Thirst drive: The tissues of the body lose fluid when fluids have not been taken in. As a result, the mucous membranes of the throat become dry and cause sensation of thirst.

Respiratory drive: It is the drive for air or oxygen. One cannot survive for long without a regular supply of air or oxygen. If oxygen is not supplied even for a short time, it is possible to experience brain damage, loss of memory and control over one's body functions.

Sleep drive: It is usually occurs at regular intervals for each person. When the body continues activities without rest or sleep for a long time, it is possible to experience confusion, inability to pay attention, droopy eyelids, staring, muscle tremors and increased sensitivity to pain. The body temperature and metabolism drop enough during sleep, saving up energy.

Drive for elimination of wastes: When the bladder or intestine become distended with waste material, they cause pressure and discomfort. The person becomes restless until the waste materials are disposed off and pressure relieved.

Sex drive: It is considered a biological drive, since it is dependent on physiological conditions. Unlike hunger and thirst, sex is not essential for the survival of the individual but is necessary for the survival of the species.

The initial drive to sex activity comes from nervous tensions within the body set up by sex hormones. Its expression is subject to moral codes and civil law. We have to sublimate sex drive by engaging ourselves with art and painting, creative writing, dramatics, etc.

Maternal drive: Maternal behaviour is instinctive in nature. It is unlearned. Physiological drive causes maternal behaviour. Maternal drive is caused by prolactin, a hormone secreted by the pituitary.

Social/Learned/Secondary Motives

Human beings are not only biological but also social. Therefore, human behaviour is activated by the following social motives:

- Achievement motives
- Affiliation motives
- Aggression motives
- Power motives
- Curiosity motives.

These are called social motives because they develop through relationship with people.

Theories of Motivation

1. McClelland's Achievement Theory

The need for achievement: Achievement motivation refers to a drive towards some standard of excellence. People with high need for achievement prefer tasks that would promise success and are moderately difficult. David C McClelland has found that while high achievers tend to succeed, low achievers tend to avoid failures. High achievers challenge failures and work harder while low achievers accept failures and go for less difficult tasks. High achievers prefer personal responsibility and like to get feedback about their work.

Children whose parents have accepted their independence tend to become high achievers. Children of overprotective parents become low achievers. Children learn by copying the behaviour of their parents and other significant people who serve as models. Through such observational learning, children adopt the characteristics of the model, including the need for achievement. The expectations that the parents have for their children also develop achievement motivation in children.

Affiliation motives: Man cannot exist in isolation. The need to be with other people is referred to as affiliation need. This need is revealed by a need to be attached to others through friendship, sociability or group membership. They make more local phone calls, visits and seek approval of others. Need to rely on others which is called dependency motive is one form of the need for affiliation. When little children are frightened, they seek others to comfort them. This kind of experience in early life makes one seek the friendly company of others when faced with anxiety and fear.

Aggression motives: Intense frustration after high expectations, verbal and non-verbal insults, fear and anxiety can trigger aggression. Television and cinema depicting violence can make youngsters model themselves to aggressive behaviour.

Psychoanalysts maintain that each individual, as part of his biological inheritance, possesses destructive death urges as well as constructive life urges. In most of us, a favourable balance exists between life and death urges, so that kindness triumphs over cruelty. Social learning (modelling), classical conditioning and instrument conditioning are ways in which hostile aggression may be learned.

Power motives: Social power is defined as the ability or capacity of a person to produce intended effect on the behaviour or emotions of other people. Persons with power motives will be concerned with having impact, reputation and influence. They exercise their power by joining political parties, voluntary organisations and associating with prominent and popular men. They select jobs which have an impact on others and dominate weaker sections of the society. They often try to convince others, play more competitive sports and drink more heavily.

Need for status: Almost all individuals have a desire to have some standing or position among the people of his society or group. Nobody likes to be considered inferior. Efforts to achieve a rank in the hierarchy of the group is present not only in human beings but even among animals and birds, e.g. "pecking order" among hens.

Need for self-actualisation: Refer the humanistic theory by Maslow and Rogers described later in this chapter.

Need Deprivation

When needs are not satisfied, it is called need deprivation. Deprivation of the need to be loved makes it very difficult to express love to others. Most cases of child abuse come from parents who received no love and security in their own childhood. When deprived of the need of self-esteem or social status, people respond with tremendous frustration and aggressive harmful behaviour. Riots, violence and murder follow. Sensory deprivation or lack of stimulation through the senses cause abnormalities in behaviour. Experiments have been conducted by placing a person in an isolated room with no light or sound. The results of these experiments showed that severe sensory deprivation can cause disorientation, confusion, restlessness, irritability, emotional upsets and loss of concentration.

2. Homeostasis or Optimum-level Theory

Claud Bernard coined the word "homeostasis" to explain the stability of the inner environment or physiological equilibrium.

For example, a healthy body maintains a certain amount of water level in the body, certain degree of body temperature and a constant rate of blood pressure. The amount of sugar in the blood should be optimal. In an attempt to maintain an internal physiological balance, the body tries to regulate itself. This process is automatic in nature and the maintenance of balance they attain is referred to as homeostasis. For example, the heat of a summer day makes one perspire and often drink water to avoid dehydration. A cold winter night makes one shiver and speed up the rate of metabolism. This brings about more heat as shivering burns the body's fuel faster and thus produce more heat. Similar deprivation of food or water causes a physiological imbalance and only consumption of food or water can bring about a balance.

3. Humanistic Theory by Abraham Maslow and Carl Rogers

Humanistic theory states that human behaviour is motivated by creativity and self-motivation. Abraham Maslow (1908–1970) classified motives into five categories and arranged them in a hierarchical fashion. Basic biological needs form the base of this hierarchy. In an ascending order, the five needs are arranged according to their importance. They are:

1. Physiological motives (hunger, thirst, etc.)
2. Safety needs (protection from harm or injury)
3. Love needs (affection, warmth, belongingness)
4. Esteem needs (self-respect, self-approval)
5. Self-actualisation (achieving maximum development of one's potential).

Motivation is based on both physiological and psychological factors. The needs at one level should be at least partially-satisfied before the needs at the next level become active. For example, when food and safety are difficult to obtain, the satisfaction of these needs will dominate a person's actions and the higher motives (growth or learned needs) will not have any significance. Only when the biological needs are satisfied to an adequate level, the individual will have the time and energy for aesthetic and intellectual pursuits. If the social needs are not satisfied, it will cause mental tension leading to psychic disorders. The need in the highest level of hierarchy is the need for self-actualisation. Self-actualisation is the ultimate goal of life. This is the need for the fullest development of one's potential and achieve something spectacular. It means achieving all one is capable of achieving (Fig. 3.1).

4. Psychoanalytic Theory by Sigmund Freud (Unconscious Motivation)

Motivation is due to a combination of biological factors, external forces and unconscious phenomenon.

Our actions are determined by the inner forces or impulses, often operating below the level of consciousness. Freud believed that all behaviour stemmed from two opposing groups of instincts, the life instincts (Eros) that enhance life and the death instincts (Thanatos) that push towards destruction. Activities to satisfy hunger, thirst, sex, etc. are life instincts. Activities to satisfy aggression and destructive tendencies are death instincts. Life activities are interaction of life and death instincts. The energy of

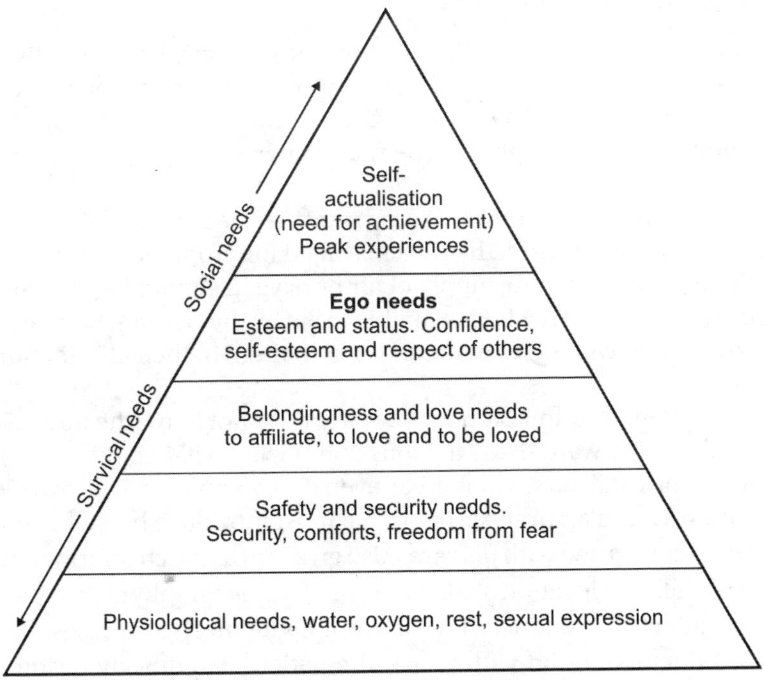

Fig. 3.1: Maslow's hierarchy of needs

the life instinct is the libido which involves mainly sex and related activities. The death instincts can be directed inwards in the form of suicide or self-destructive behaviour or outwards in the form of aggression towards others.

Freud also emphasised the powerful role of unconscious motives in human behaviour. He pointed to several forms of behaviour through which unconscious motives are expressed:

a. In dreams, we often express wishes and impulses of which we are unaware.
b. Unconscious mannerisms, slips of pen and tongue, our irrational fears of specific objects or phobias reveal hidden motives.
c. Our chronic headaches, insomnia, gastric troubles for which there are no physical or organic reasons, show the unconscious needs of the person.

Motivation and the Nurse

The nurse has to remember that motives are at work in the lives of patients, colleagues and her own daily relationships. Understanding own motives and motives in the patient will help the nurse to build a cooperative relationship between the patient and the health care team.

The nurse should always be aware of the need for the satisfaction of the primary needs. The patient's need for proper food, water or fluids and a constant supply of air or oxygen should be met. She must feed patients who are unable to eat by themselves. Similarly, cover them with blankets and also help them in their elimination needs.

Patient, on admission to the ward, does not know the do's and don'ts in the ward. He is anxious about what will happen to him. In uniform, all nurses look alike, even though uniform will provide authority and assurance. The nurse must introduce herself as the nurse concerned with his care. Also give him as much information especially the location of toilets and general geography of the ward. A regular ward routine, with fixed timings for meals, drugs, visitors' and doctors' round with which the patient can quickly become familiar also will add to security. Patients should be helped to retain intact their family and social links. For small children, it is particularly important that the bond with their parents remains intact.

Relatives and friends demonstrate their love and affection by bringing flowers and presents and by sending cards and letters. These symbolic acts should be treated with respect by the nursing staff. The nurse's help may be needed during visiting time to ensure privacy.

The very fact that one has fallen ill and is unable to work or cope with the home and family is a threat to self-esteem. The stigma attached to certain illnesses like tuberculosis and leprosy and to certain types of hospitals like cancer hospitals adds to this problem. It may not be possible to avoid all the practices known to lower self-esteem, e.g. asking a patient to undress and expose his body for physical examination, but nurses should recognise that this is humiliating to the patients, and therefore, should be minimum.

It is particularly distressing to the adolescent who has only recently established his independence to have his bodily needs attended to by nurses who are not much older than himself. Nurse should restrain from "talking down" to patients when giving instructions or information. The nurse should avoid intrusive history-taking and should keep all information strictly confidential.

There is a skill involved in conveying to a patient unconditional respect and acceptance when his sickness has reduced his value as a human being.

Though it is difficult for the nurse to contribute to the self-actualisation needs of patients, she should remember that some patients discover their artistic, literary or musical talent through various forms of art and occupational therapy. Patients may have "peak experiences" or heightened religious faith through suffering, tragedy and a contemplation of impending death.

QUESTIONS

1. Describe the nature and the biological basis of motivation.
2. Write short notes on:

a. Needs of patients and nurses
b. Human motivation
c. Drive
d. Homeostasis
e. Self-actualisation
f. Self-esteem
g. Need deprivation.

3. Explain human motivation. How are motives classified? What is the importance of motivation in patient care?
4. Describe any two theories of motivation.

4 Frustration and Conflicts

Motivation is an internal urge to act towards a particular goal. When motives are hindered or blocked, frustration occurs. People who cannot achieve their important goals feel depressed, anxious, fearful, guilty or angry (Fig. 4.1).

Frustration is a negative feeling when one is prevented from reaching a goal. For example, one will be frustrated if:

a. After getting up early to bathe before most others, one finds that there is no water.
b. After studying very hard, one fails in the examination.

Sources of Frustration

1. *Environmental forces* (external sources) that block motive fulfilment. The obstacle may be something physical, e.g. a locked door, lack of money or it may be people—parents, teachers or policemen. The restrictions placed on behaviour by the rules of the society is another source of frustration.
2. *Personal inadequacies* (internal sources) that make it impossible to reach goals. For example, some people are handicapped by blindness or paralysis. As children grow into adulthood, the

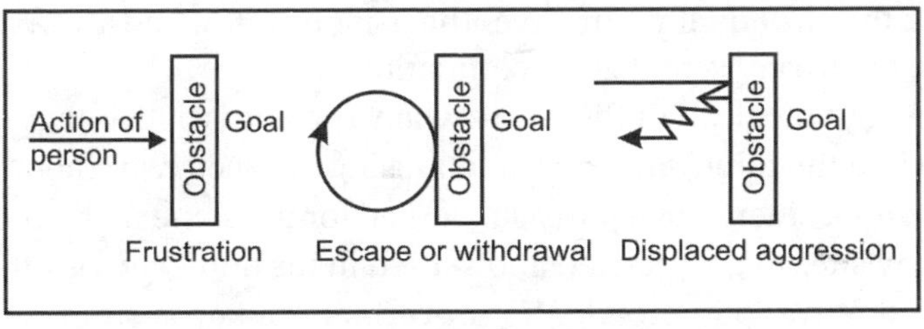

Fig. 4.1: Frustration leads to aggression

unattainable goals bring more and more frustration. These are mainly learned goals that cannot be achieved because they are beyond the person's abilities. A boy may learn to aspire for too high an academic achievement but is neither very intelligent nor hard-working. He gets only low marks because of his level of performance.

Most individuals have somewhat similar desires, but they are not equally equipped to satisfy them. In life's struggle for health, marital partners and other values, the more gifted encounter less obstacles than the less endowed. All things being equal, some perform better than the less privileged.

3. *Conflict between motives:* The most serious and deep-rooted frustration occurs due to conflict between motives. Conflict is like a tug of war between two or more courses of action or opposing ideas. The person is required to act one way or the other often generating painful emotions. Conflict is a special type of frustration. The existence of frustration in life is unavoidable, without which development is not possible. When conflicts become excessive they become harmful. Excessive conflicts indicate a weakness of determination. Strong will power is needed to overcome conflicts. These conflicts are of four basic forms. In each of these conflicts, attainment of a goal, for a time, is hindered. Depending on the type of conflict, various emotional and behavioural reactions may occur.

Types of Conflicts

Conflicts are of four basic forms:

Approach-Approach Conflict (Fig. 4.2)

This is the simplest kind of conflict and occurs between two positive goals that are equally attractive. The person is attracted at the same time by two goals that are incompatible.

A physiological conflict arises when a person is both hungry and sleepy at the same time, such as choosing between two cinemas or to go for a cinema or a party scheduled for the same night. A man who wishes to get married and settled in his homeland is offered an attractive job abroad. The proverbial donkey is supposed to

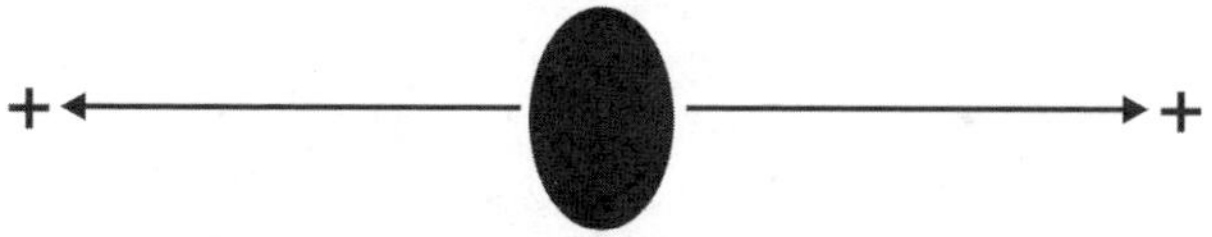

Fig. 4.2: Approach-approach conflict

have starved to death because it stood halfway between two piles of hay and could not decide which to eat first.

When one is able to make up one's mind quickly and easily, the conflict is resolved. Even more serious approach-approach conflicts, such as choosing your place of work after graduation can be resolved more quickly than other types of conflicts.

Avoidance-Avoidance Conflict (Fig. 4.3)

It takes place when you are forced to choose between two negative goals. An individual is caught between the devil and the deep blue sea because of personal needs and moral values. The individual is caught between two threats, fears or situations that are equally repelling. One has to choose between toothache and going to the dentist. One may dislike studies and also failure and has to choose between the two. Another avoidance conflict is between unhappy employment and loss of income. These conflicts are not resolved quickly but often go on for a long time.

An example of an avoidance conflict which reflects one's personal belief is having to choose between abortion and unwanted pregnancy. Another example is jumping down from a burning building.

The avoidance conflict is the worst type of conflict and is stressful. It leads to indecision, vacillation, inaction and sometimes "freezing" and "escape"—leaving the field (suicide) (vertical arrow in Figure 4.3).

Theoretically, a person might escape the avoidance conflict by running away from the field and people try this. In practice, however, there are additional negative forces in the periphery of the situation that prevent them from running away. For example, a girl who does not want either to do her arithmetic or get a spanking

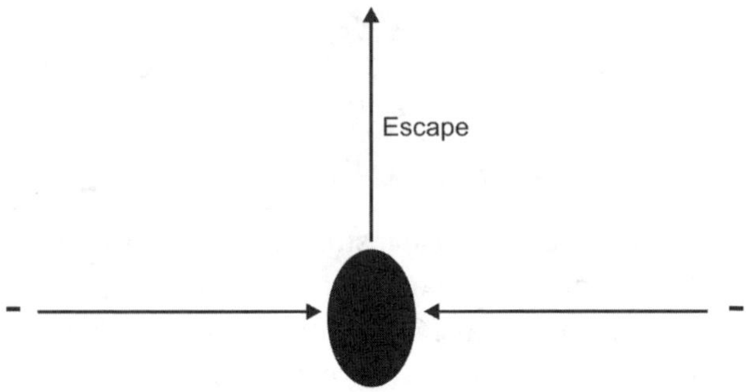

Fig. 4.3: Avoidance-avoidance conflict

might think of running away from home. But the consequences of running away are even worse than her other alternatives, and so she does not do it. A man must have preventive surgery or run the risk of later illness.

People in avoidance-avoidance conflicts, may try different means of running away. They often rely on imagination to free them from the fear and anxiety generated by the conflict. They may spend much of their time in day-dreaming, conjuring up an imaginary world where there are no conflicts or they may recreate in their minds the carefree world of their childhood before the unpleasant tasks and avoidance-avoidance conflict existed. This way of leaving the conflict is called regression.

Approach-Avoidance Conflict (Fig. 4.4)

It is the most difficult to resolve because in this conflict, a person is both attracted and repelled by the same goal (object). We speak of ambivalance as the person has positive and negative feelings about the same event.

Ice cream is delicious but also causes obesity. A man wants to marry a girl for her beauty but at the same time her educational level is too low. A girl wants parental protection but at the same time does not want parental domination. A child wants to pat a dog but is afraid and pulls back his hand. A person picks up the

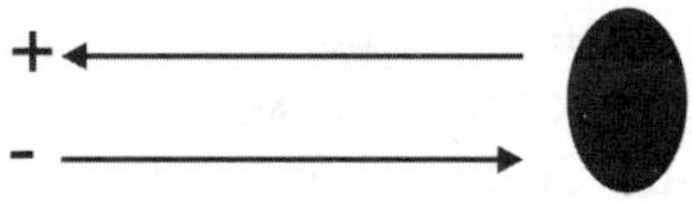

Fig. 4.4: Approach-avoidance conflict

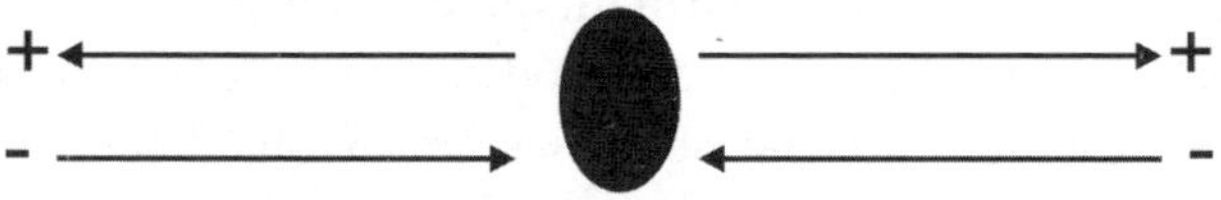

Fig. 4.5: Double approach-avoidance conflict

telephone and dials a number, but fearing other person's response, puts the receiver back.

Multiple Approach-Avoidance Conflicts (Fig. 4.5)

Many of life's problems involve many positive and many negative goals.

Consider the student who experiences a conflict between making good grades and making it to the college football team. Superficially, this appears to be a simple case of approach-approach conflict, between two positive goals. But the obedient boy experiences considerable social pressures from his family and friends to achieve both the goals. He may incur the disapproval of his parents if he fails to make good grades in studies. He will lose the esteem of his friends if he does not make it to the college football team. Failure at either end carries a threat.

Another example is, a career woman engaged to be married. The goal of marriage has a positive value for her because of the stability and security it will provide and because she loves the man she will be marrying. But marriage is repellent to her because it will mean giving up an attractive offer of job in another city. If the over-all sum of marriage values is greater than that of the career, she might hesitate for a while, vacillate back and forth, and then get married.

In still another example, a man may be in conflict not only about whether to get married but also about which of the several girls would make the ideal wife. Internal obstacles are harder to resolve than the external ones.

People may find ways to getting around environmental obstacles but they find it very hard to escape from obstacles within themselves, i.e. from personal inadequacies and conflicts between motives. The emotional reactions due to approach-avoidance conflicts in which internal obstacles are involved cause several behavioural problems. Conflicts are resolved through the use of certain methods of thinking and acting which either eliminate the conflict or reduce its severity.

Reactions to Frustrations

Frustration creates uncomfortable emotional tensions and so the individual tries to reduce the tension in a variety of ways. The important reactions are as follows:

Direct approach: Two direct methods of overcoming obstacles are increased effort and changing the mode of attack. If both the methods fail, the third alternative is in changing the goal to one that is more attainable.

Feelings of inferiority: When increased effort and variation of attack fail and substitute goals are unavailable, individual often react by developing feelings of helplessness and inadequacy. This emotionally distressing state of the mind is referred to as inferiority complex. An inferiority complex is the form of self-criticism usually involving fear of social disapproval. The common reactions are fear of competition, extreme sensitivity to criticism, suspicion, envy, self-consciousness, worry and extreme self-analysis.

Aggressiveness: Instead of adjusting passively to obstacles with a defeatist attitude, many react aggressively towards the source of frustration. Aggressive reaction is very common when some external obstacle is the cause of frustration. The target of attack is usually some other person or object and the intensity of attack is proportionate to the amount of frustration.

Coping with Frustration and Conflict

Frustration and conflict cause stress and anxiety causing harm to the body. Some common reactions to frustrations are persistence, escape and aggression. Some methods of relieving frustration are:

1. Identify the source of your frustration. Can you change it or control it. If you cannot, learning to accept the situation might be the right answer.
2. Decide important things carefully. Check everything out carefully before making a change in your job or residence.
3. Try to find compromises. Look for positive things when all choice seem negative.
4. Seek reliable help from advisors, teachers and other counsellors.
5. Avoid indecision. Stick to your decision and forget about the other choices unless you are clearly wrong.

QUESTIONS

1. What are the different kinds of conflicts?
2. Define frustration and conflict. Discuss different types of conflicts. Write about any two conflicts that you have experienced and resolved in your present training.
3. How are frustration and conflict related to each other? Show how you can handle conflict situations in the best possible way.
4. Which of the social motives are likely to be frustrated in a chronically ill patient? Give two suitable examples to show what you can do to help a person to overcome frustration in a healthy way.
5. "Three basic types of conflicts arise from incompatible motives" What are they and how do they arise? How can your knowledge about the nature of conflicts help you in your profession?

5 Defence Mechanisms or Adjustment Mechanisms

Adjustment Mechanisms or Defence Mechanism

Freud, in 1904, used the term "defence mechanism" to refer to the unconscious process that defends a person against anxiety. When the primitive ID drives are in serious conflict with the controls imposed by the *'Ego'* or the *'Superego'*, the individual suffers from tension and anxiety. This uncomfortable situation is reflected in the individual's behaviour. Some method of developing a compromise and relieving the tension and anxiety is needed. The human being is usually able to reduce the tension by utilising certain forms of adaptation which are called ego defence mechanisms, adjustment mechanisms or mental dynamisms.

Defence mechanisms enable a person to "resolve the conflict" and reduce the "stress and anxiety" associated with it. Of course, many of these strategies are self-deceptive in nature. When more adaptive measures to resolve the conflicts are not available to the individual, these mechanisms help him to live comfortably without having to face very difficult problems. For instance, individuals who suffer from a disease such as cancer and are sure to die, may deny such a state of affairs to themselves and may plan their future projects as if they have many years of life before them. Such a denial of fact rids the individual of the agony of thinking about his impending death.

Mental mechanisms are a means of compromising with forbidden desires, feelings of guilt or an admission that one is inadequate in facing certain problems. They salvage the individual's self-respect, avoid an open admission of failure and save psychic energy. With the exception of sublimation, all defence mechanisms indicate an inner conflict.

All of us use defence mechanisms some time or the other in our normal behaviour. When used moderately, they are harmless and help us face, conflicts and frustrations easily and protect our ego. However, excessive and persistent use of these mechanisms is harmful as they do not solve conflicts and frustrations basically, but only help the individual to make adaptations to distressing experiences.

Defence mechanisms can be divided into successful and unsuccessful mechanisms as given below:

Successful	*Unsuccessful*
Repression	Suppression
Rationalisation	Reaction formation
Intellectualisation	Displacement
Compensation	Denial
Substitution	Isolation
Sublimation	Projection
	Regression
	Conversion
	Fixation
	Fantasy

Repression

According to Freud, repression is basic to all other forms of defence mechanisms. Repression refers to the process by which an individual strives to keep unacceptable, painful, unpalatable and anxiety provoking needs, urges and feelings associated with them in the unconscious layers of the mind. The occurrence of the process of repression is itself unconscious, and hence the individual is unaware of such urges. We forget and then forget that we forgot.

When we cast a discomforting idea or desire deliberately out of our mind or field of attention, we call it suppression. Suppressed material is easily recalled and is, thus, available to the conscious mind.

When this process takes place unconsciously, we call it repression. A group of repressed desires and ideas, strongly emotionally toned, forms a complex.

In terms of psychic energy, repression is an expensive defence mechanism. If it operates smoothly and prevents feelings of anxiety, it may help promote a well adjusted life. However, it is a sort of "burying alive" mechanism. The repressed material is always active and the unconscious memories or urges continue to seek expression and may emerge in the form of accidents" (e.g. "slips of the tongue or pen") or neurotic symptoms. Many painful experiences are repressed during early childhood and become unconscious sources of emotional conflict in later life. Selfish, hostile feelings and sexual impulses are frequently repressed. These may later escape through conversion into obsessions and into morbid anxiety that arises without apparent reason.

Repression is a process of unconscious forgetfulness of our unpleasant and conflict producing emotions and desires. If these experiences were to remain in the conscious, they would cause a person to feel ashamed, guilty and unworthy. For example:

1. People may forget to turn up for an appointment for a treatment they do not like.
2. Mistakes made in nursing patients may be forgotten.

The repressed material forms part of the unconscious level of the mind and may affect behaviour without the person being aware (unconscious motivation). For example, a child may feel angry with his mother because she had punished him. If he feels too guilty about his anger, he may repress it and may still be unconsciously angry. This may be shown by the accidental breaking of his mother's favourite things or in his bed wetting or refusal of food.

Reaction Formation

It is sometimes possible to conceal a motive from ourselves by giving strong expression to its opposite. Such a tendency is called reaction formation. The mother of an unwanted child may feel guilty and so becomes over indulgent and over-protective of the child to assure herself that she is a good overtly mother.

People who are extremely friendly, overtly polite and very socially correct, frequently have unconscious feelings of anger and hatred towards many people.

Another example is the mother-in-law—daughter-in-law problem. Daughter-in-law talks very highly of her mother-in-law and vice versa.

Projection

Projection is a frequently used unconscious mechanism that relieves tension and anxiety by transferring the responsibility for unacceptable ideas, impulses, wishes or thoughts to another person. It is an attempt to deal with our own shortcomings, by seeing them in others and denying them in ourselves.

The student who believes that everybody cheats in examinations may also cheat in the same way. People who are dishonest often attribute dishonesty to others. An adulterer blames his wife that she is an adulteress. When we feel guilty about our dislike of another nurse, we complain that she is the one who dislikes us. The nurse who is poor in clinical practice may claim that all health care team members are giving poor patient care. The surgeon who bungled an operation may insist that it happened because the theatre nurse and ward boy did their task poorly. Carried to the extreme, projection is the mask of a behaviour disorder known as paranoia.

When you practice projection, your relationship with others will be strained. Firstly, you will not see or understand your own failings. Secondly, you will find others relating poorly with you because of your negative attitude towards them. Thirdly, you will find it very difficult to accept responsibilities for your own behaviour because you blame others for anything that goes wrong.

Rationalisation

In rationalisation, we "make excuses" giving a reason different from the real one for what we are doing. It is a defence mechanism in which an individual justifies his failures and socially unacceptable behaviours by giving socially approved reasons. For example, students who fail in the examination may complain that the hostel atmosphere was not favourable for study. A tense father who beats his child may rationalise that it is for the child's good. A scientist who is unable to carry out research of high order may blame the lack of facilities in his laboratory. An employee who fails to get promotion may blame the employer's partiality.

Rationalisation is not lying. We believe in our explanations. It is like a blanket to cover the human weaknesses. It operates in two forms:

a. Sour grapes, and
b. Sweet lemon.

Sour grape (from Aesop's fable of the fox and grapes): A young man who fails to get a beautiful wife may remark that a beautiful wife is a liability. A doctor without a vehicle "does not want to risk his life" by driving a scooter or a car. A girl who fails to get admission for the nursing course may point out a number of difficulties of the nursing profession. "An unskilled worker always quarrels about his tools".

Sweet lemon form is an extension of the "sour grape" type. The individual justifies his lower achievements by pointing out their merits. For example, a poor, idle man "does not want to earn more money" because "money is the root cause of many evils". People living in small houses due to limited financial resources may point out many virtues of small houses. A husband who fails to get a highly educated wife may also enumerate a number of virtues in an uneducated woman.

Intellectualisation

Related to rationalisation is intellectualisation, another defence mechanism which involves reasoning. It is the distancing from an emotional or threatening situation by talking or thinking about it in intellectual terms. A nurse, doctor or paramedical worker cannot afford to becoome emotionally attached to each patient. So they use the technique of detaching themselves from emotions through calm abstract statements about the situation. As a student nurse, probably you use this most of the time when working with patients who are acutely or terminally ill. You may speak calmly and intelligently rather than emotionally with patients and their families. For example, if there is a patient who is acutely ill, calmly tell the family members rather than saying "I am so sorry", etc.

This is a helpful defence mechanism to separate yourself from professional crises. But to go on using it in all your relationships and experiences is to become a very cold and detached individual without healthy emotional experiences.

Displacement

Displacement means to substitute the real object of one's feelings which are often aggression, with another object. A person who is angry with his boss, but cannot show it for fear of losing the job may fight with his wife and children on return from the office or kick his dog. Anger against the ward sister may be displaced on to a more junior nurse or a patient. When a new baby is the centre of attraction, an older child may become jealous; prevented from harming the baby, the child demolishes a doll.

Regression

To regress in behaviour means to behave in a less mature way, i.e. go backwards. An adult behaving like a child is practising regression. When faced with difficulties of life, an individual reverts to a less mature form of behaviour, where he finds less conflict, and hence less anxiety.

Faced with the unwelcome arrival of a new baby or going to school for the first time, a five years old may have toilet accidents, revert to "baby talk", demand cuddling, etc. "Crying on someone's shoulder" is symbolic of the infant's seeking comfort at the maternal bosom. You may practice regression when faced with pressures of an examination. Another example is, when the nurse makes an error in giving medicines or nursing care and then starts crying.

Adults too, may regress to the oral stage of development and suck their thumbs when life gets stressful. One may regress so profoundly that he will curl up in the fetal position and remain in it without moving. Any retreat into a state of dependency or other to avoid facing acute problems is called a regressive trait.

Some regressions, such as tears on becoming very emotional are quite normal while facing serious problems in life. Extreme forms and degrees of regression result in psychosis.

Sublimation

It is the channelling of a strong and socially unacceptable drive or urge into a form that is acceptable to society. The most important of these are sexual desires. Others are aggressive feeling, greed and even lying.

Sublimation is one of the more positive mechanisms of adjustment and is responsible for much of the artistic and cultural achievements of the civilised people. An unmarried woman can express repressed sexual desires, by becoming a nursery school teacher. A young man who has lost his lover may turn to write poetry about love. A person who has aggressive feelings may not be able to express these in society but can become a boxer or soldier. A person with greed can become a successful businessman. A person who needs love can re-channel these energies into fiction writing.

The unfulfilled need to give maternal care may find gratification in the care of the sick. Some lonely people give much love and care to cats and dogs when no opportunity occurs for giving their affection to human beings. One positive result of sublimation is personal satisfaction experienced by the individual. Society also profits as activities like creative writing, music, painting and sculpturing as a result of sublimation are enjoyed.

Identification

By this adjustment, the individual feels the personal satisfaction in the success and achievements of other people and groups. Thus, the little boy takes the masculine attributes that he admires in his father. Girls identify with their mother, later perhaps with their teacher, and later still perhaps with a film star. Young nurses identify with the ward sister. Hero worship is an obvious form of identification.

Parents may identify themselves with their children. An illiterate father often takes his son's higher education as his own achievement. A dignified mother takes her daughter's failures as her own degeneration. Many people, while watching a film identify with the hero and heroine to the extent that they burst into tears when the hero/heroine is shown mercilessly attacked by villains.

Much of the learning process in childhood is through identification. As we grow a little older, we identify with our teachers, legendary figures, heroes, idols and icons.

A very common age for practising identification is the teens. Adolescents often identify with successful people in the movies. Identification with a hero either in fiction or in real life is called hero-worship.

Identification is quite normal and healthy, since it plays a large part in the development of a child's personality and in the process of acculturation. Through the process of identification, a child takes on the desirable attributes found in the personalities of people in his environment for whom he has admiration and affection. If the object with which we identify is good, their effect on us will be constructive; if it is bad, the effect can be destructive. Also, we cannot grow and mature if we are completely satisfied by identifying with the experiences and successes of others. We must have our own identify for our growth.

Compensation

Compensation means something given to replace a loss or to make up for a defect. Just as nature compensates for disease in our bodies (as when a blind person develops extraordinarily keen hearing), so we develop personality traits to compensate for various inadequacies. When people are frustrated in their desires in one direction, they compensate for it by attaining success in other directions. A student who fails in his studies may compensate by becoming the college champion in athletics. A plain girl who cannot compete with her more beautiful sisters may compensate by studying hard and come first in her class. Rivalry often leads to compensation. A mother is over-protective of and over-indulgent to a child whom unconsciously she rejects. When carried to excess, it is called over compensation. Students practice compensation when they excel in objective and practical exams after doing poorly in eassy type questions. Helen Keller was born blind and deaf but her determination overcame these handicaps and she won world fame. Cosmologist Stephen Hawking even though on Wheelchair and not able to speak, is a top scientist in Cambridge University.

Denial

Denial of reality is when we refuse to accept or believe in the existence of something that is very unpleasant to us. We use denial most often when faced with death, serious illness or something painful and threatening. A patient often practices denial, at least for a period of time, when he knows he has a fatal illness but cannot accept his impending death. Parents of fatally ill children will also deny the serious nature of illness for some time. Many old people will not easily accept that their mental and physical powers are on the decline as they advance in age. Backward students do not find any reliability in the intelligence tests. When some very near and dear one dies in the family, some people try to keep up the pretence that he is still alive. At the dining table, his place is left empty. A patient admitted to the psychiatric ward may say that he just "needs rest." A student who spends beyond his means is denying his lack of money. Often, nurses protect themselves from the impact of the numerous traumatic experiences of emergencies, suffering and death by developing an unfeeling and apparently callous attitude.

Denial is quite harmless if practised in moderation, but can lead to serious difficulties in health and lifestyle if practised to excess.

Fantasy or Daydreaming

It is a kind of withdrawal when faced with real problems of life. We retire to a make belief world, where everything is possible, where we are victors or conquerors. The tendency to daydreaming is most pronounced during adolescence.

Daydreaming is a pleasant thing. It may help us to escape during times of stress. For example, when one is having financial problems, one can escape from them temporarily by planning how to spend an imaginary fortune. Patients who are very ill may fantasise that when they recover, many good things will happen to them.

Fantasy may offer temporary relief from pressures. But excessive daydreaming may lead to loss of contact with realities and may lead to a psychotic disorder called schizophrenia.

Withdrawal

Whenever an individual suspects that he is likely to be criticised, ridiculed or disgraced on account of some prior unfortunate experience or failure, he resorts to withdrawal. Such a person is seen as avoiding all work saying that he cannot do this or that. It is a protective device by which the individual prevents further hurt and damage to his security by withdrawing from people and avoding all close interpersonal relations. It may occur as a temporary pattern. They make no real friends.

Withdrawal is one of the dominant personality traits of the schizophrenics. These patients not only have an inability to relate well with people emotionally but they also use "regression."

Conversion

Conversion is a defence mechanism by which an emotional conflict is expressed as a physical symptom for which there is no demonstrable organic basis. A student nurse, very anxious about her exam, may develop a headache. A woman invited for a party which presents an upsetting situation to her, develop gastrointestinal symptoms and may excuse herself from the party. Usually when the party time is over, her symptoms resolve themselves.

Conversion hysteria is the converting of strong emotional conflicts into such physical symptoms that the very helplessness of the victim will resolve the conflict. For example, a soldier in the battlefield may be deeply upset at the prospect of having to kill or be killed. He develops paralysis of his legs as an unconscious defence mechanism.

Another example of this mechanism would be that of a small boy who hated his father so deeply that he wished to strike him.

He could suddenly develop complete paralysis of his right arm which would do two things for him:

a. Resolve the conflict (he cannot strike his father even if wished to do so).
b. Bring him a great deal of attention and sympathy.

Suppression

Suppression is intentional pushing away from awareness of certain unwelcome ideas, memories or feelings. We merely push them into the background, into our subconscious mind, where they are accessible to us whenever we wish to remember them. Because it is conscious, it is not a defence mechanism in the strict sense of the term. For example, a student consciously decides not to think about her weekend, so that she can study effectively. A patient may refuse to consider his difficulties by saying that he does not want to talk about it. Suppression is easier to deal with, because the material remains conscious.

Defence Mechanisms and the Nurse

Understanding defence mechanisms will enable the nurse to support the patient and his family. For example, denial is a common reaction to a serious diagnosis or at the time of death. The patient and his family should be allowed to deny the situation until they are prepared to face the reality. The patient will often practice regression through tears, trembling or demanding special treatment. Some patients may also practice withdrawal and should be allowed to do so. Many patients intellectualise about a serious sickness or prognosis just like the nurses and other members of the health team (Table 5.1).

Identification can be seen in patients who rely heavily on the nurse's advice and support. They expect that all of their needs will be met and that nothing will be expected of them. It is important for the nurse to recognise that identification can be used constructively to teach proper health care.

Patients who must deal with the stress of serious illness may shift the blame for their condition into the nurse (projection).

Table 5.1: Summary of definitions of defence mechanisms

Mechanisms	*Definition*
Repression	Unconsciously forgetting unpleasant experiences
Reaction formation	Strongly expressing the reverse of what one feels
Projection	Pretending that others have your own failings
Rationalisation	Making excuses, giving a reason different from the real one for what we are doing
Intellectualisation	Distancing oneself from emotional situations by abstract talking or thinking
Displacement	Discharging pent-up feelings on persons less dangerous than those who initially aroused the emotion
Regression	Acting immaturely
Sublimation	Directing unacceptable desires into socially acceptable behaviour
Identification	Finding satisfaction through what another person does
Compensation	Working hard to make up for a weakness or deficiency
Denial	Refusing to believe that something unpleasant exists
Fantasy	Withdrawal to a make belief world when faced with real problems
Withdrawal	Avoiding all close interpersonal relationship
Conversion	An emotional conflict is expressed by a physical illness or a physical symptom without any organic cause
Suppression	Intentional pushing away from awareness of certain unwelcome ideas, memories and feelings

They may complain of poor nursing care to a nurse who is actually very skilful. Nurses should not show anger and retaliate but should encourage the patients to explore the realistic aspects of their situation.

Both well-adjusted and maladjusted individuals make use of the decence mechanisms for their daily life. The well adjusted individuals use them sparingly and in socially desirable ways, whereas the maladjusted individuals including psychotics and neurotics use them too frequently and inappropriately.

QUESTIONS

1. Define "mental mechanisms." Name ten mental mechanisms and describe any two of them in detail.
2. Name the ego defence mechanism involved in the following:
   a. Demanding extreme degrees of health care for patients whom you always disliked.
   b. Excelling in drama when weak in studies.
   c. Saying you are fine when you are in severe pain.
   d. Staying in your room when your friends are at a party.
   e. Pretending that everybody is a liar.
   f. Daydreaming about being the best student in the science class.
   g. Forgetting that you failed in the fifth standard.
   h. Excelling in orphanage work when unmarried.
   i. Dressing up like a popular film star.
   j. Crying or pouting when you make an error.
   k. Arguing with a junior student when angry with the principal.
   l. Studying very hard after your classes are over.
   m. Believe or pretend to believe that psychology is not important.
   n. Cultivate the friendship of the best student of science.
   o. Without working hard, bask in the best student's reflected glory.
   p. Blame the lecturer for not being able to teach well or to arouse interest in the subject.
   q. Become ill or feel sick and cut classes and tests.
   r. Saying "I don't like the prize anyway" when failing to win a prize.
3. Explain:
   a. The similarities and differences between suppression and repression.
   b. How alcoholism and drugs are forms of defence mechanisms (escapism)?

6 Emotions in Health and Disease

Emotion and motivation have the same Latin origin. The Latin word '*emovere*' means to be "stirred up." Anger, fear, surprise, 'joy, grief, love, affection, hope, anticipation, acceptance, disappointment, jealousy and disgust are classified as emotion while hunger, thirst and fatigue are motives. Emotions are usually aroused by external stimuli and emotional expression is directed towards the stimuli in the environment that arouses it. Motives on the other hand are aroused by internal stimuli and are directed towards certain objects in the environment, e.g. food, water.

We often think ourselves as rational beings who go about satisfying our motives in an intelligent way. To a certain extent we do that, but we are also emotional beings, more emotional than we often realise. Life would be drab without emotions. Emotions add colour and spice to life.

Emotions and feelings are interchangeably used by many. Emotions are the outward expressions of feelings. Feelings persist for longer time than emotions. Feelings are simple and sensory. Emotions are more complex. Emotions are aroused not only by existing circumstances but also by a recollection of these circumstances.

Emotion is a strong feeling. It is a conscious stirred up state of the organism. Emotion is a disturbed grandular and muscular activity. It increases energy mobilisation. Emotion is defined as a subjective response that is usually accompanied by a physiological change and is associated with a change in behaviour.

Internal Changes in Emotion (Physiological changes in strong emotions)

The autonomic nervous system has two subdivisions—the sympathetic division and the parasympathetic division. The sympathetic division of the autonomic nervous system prepares the body for emergency action during aroused states. The sympathetic system causes discharge of hormones, epinephril (adrenaline) and norepinephril (noradrenaline). Adrenaline gets circulated to different parts of the body through blood and is responsible for the following physical changes:

a. Increase in blood pressure and heart rate.
b. Changes in the rate of respiration. When excited, breath comes in short quick gasps. When depressed, breathing is slow.
c. Dilation of pupils.
d. Sweating and decreased secretion of saliva.
e. Increase in blood glucose.
f. Production of more energy.
g. Increased mobility of the gastrointestinal tract.
h. Errect hair on the skin (goose pimples).
i. Changes in the frequency of the brain waves.
j. Muscular tensions and tremors.

Tremors are usually produced when opposing muscles are contracted simultaneously. They also occur when a person is experiencing severe conflicting desires. The parasympathetic system controls the heart rate, breathing and other vital functions when not in crisis situations, i.e. normal situations. The sympathetic and parasympathetic systems balance each other.

Polygraph: Lie Detector

The physiological changes accompanying intense emotions are the basis of the use of polygraph commonly known as the "lie detector" in checking the reliability of an individual's statement. The term "lie detector" is actually incorrect. The polygraph does not detect lies. It simply measures some of the physiological changes in emotion like alteration in heart rate, blood pressure, respiration and the galvanic skin response (GSR), i.e. changes in the electrical conductivity of the skin. The method is not foolproof and is not admissible in a court of law.

External Changes in Emotion

Change in the voice is experienced in many persons. Emotions like fear and excitement are expressed externally by a smile or laughter. A tremor in the voice, denotes sorrow and sharp high pitch indicates anger.

Changes in the facial expression are indicative of emotional responses. Primary emotions like interest, enjoyment, surprise, disgust, anger, shame and fear are expressed externally by facial expressions.

Changes in the different parts of the body (body language) like stiffness of the body, the way a person holds his head and the way he folds his hands are non-verbal expressions of emotions.

Body Language: Non-verbal Communication

Body language means communication through body movement such as facial expressions, postures and gestures. It is called a language because all of these movements send a message to another person along with anything that is said verbally.

Much body language is universal. Leaning towards another person or object means liking while drawing away means disliking. Smiling means pleasantness and frowning shows unpleasantness. Spitting at another person means contempt or disgust in any culture. Shaking or throwing one's shoes or sandal at another person is a sign of extreme disgust.

Fright or Flight Syndrome or Emergency Theory

Walter Cannon, the Harvard physiologist, has said that the internal changes in emotions are useful to people who must fight or flee. Cannon noted that the physical aspects of such emotions as anger or fear help the organism survive in case of danger. The adrenal glands pour out adrenaline into the blood stream and extra-strength or power is available for quick action.

Importance of Emotions

Emotions occupy a very important position in a person's life as they motivate many in their job endeavours. A person in love makes sacrifices for the object of his love. The love of their offspring spurs the parents to great sacrifices.

Emotions have a stimulating effect. For example, a person who is in a happy state of mind invariably makes others also happy and sees happiness around him. Similarly, a person who is angry makes others angry. Thus, emotion is contagious. Emotions also play a crucial role in creative and artistic activities. A soldier lays down his life for the love of his country. The ability to understand and interpret the emotional states of others is very important in our social life. It is clear that emotions play a major role in our behaviour and in understanding other's behaviour. Sometimes emotions are beneficial and at other times they are harmful. It depends on the intensity and duration of emotion. When emotion becomes intense whether pleasant or unpleasant, they usually result in some disruption of thought or behaviour. So also, when emotions are prolonged or excessive they do harm because of the sustained physiological changes that accompany them.

Emotions and Disease

Excess emotions not only have an inhibiting effect on the ability to think, but also have a permanent harmful effect on the body. Illness and excess emotions always go together. A branch of medical science has developed known as psychosomatic medicine.

Many physical complaints are related to the patient's psychological reactions to life. Peptic ulcer has its origin in emotional stresses. Colitis is caused psychosomatically. Many skin diseases, blood pressure, asthma and migraine are caused by emotional stress. Emotion can interfere with the course of a disease even when it may not be a cause of the disease. Emotions work against the successful treatment of tuberculosis, diabetes, heart diseases and epilepsy.

Emotions need not be eliminated but should be controlled. Emotion can be a major barrier to communication. The nurse should be able to understand the emotions of the patients and her own, so that she can help the patient to meet his or her needs. Once the emotional barriers are broken down, a feeling of mutual trust between the patient and the nurse develops and the patient will begin to talk more freely about himself. This is the basis of an effective nurse-patient relationship.

THE NURSE AND CONTROL OF EMOTIONS

As a nurse, you should be concerned with the expression and control of emotions:

a. In yourself
b. In others.

In Yourself

As a nurse, you are the central figure in health care. You will be much more poised and productive if you are emotionally controlled and mature in you behaviour. Emotional poise is also important for your physical and mental health. The following suggestions will help you develop emotional poise:

1. Try to understand yourself, your conflicts and your physical and emotional limits.
2. Learn as much as you can, about the causes and physical reactions to emotions. The more you know, better control over emotions.
3. Control stress in your life. Plan your work to avoid emergencies.
4. Balance your work with play, exercise and social activities.
5. Practice relaxation by meditation, listening to music, reading, dancing or sports.
6. Use your sense of humour. Laughter with others and laughing at yourself can relieve tensions in your body.
7. Try to control unreasonable and excessive external expressions of emotions. These external expressions tend to increase the intensity of emotional experiences of the individual. They excite other people and cause further emotionality.
8. A desirable philosophy of life will enable you to avoid mental conflicts and emotional tensions.

Control of Emotions in the Patients

When you first come into contact with a patient, he will respond to whatever message you give through the tone of your voice and body language.

Help the Patient Feel Welcome and at Ease

Give a warm welcome to the patient. Let him feel that he is an important guest. Let not the patient know your feelings, if any, of frustration due to the heavy work load or any negative feeling towards the patient. Your top priority at the beginning of a patient's relationship is to provide a pleasant, relaxed atmosphere.

Understand His Negative Emotions

Normally, the patients are less self-controlled than the nurses. They are tense, irritable and unbalanced. Therefore, the nurse has to be very patient, mature and balanced in her behaviour towards the patients.

Promote Positive Feelings

The nurse has to substitute the negative emotions of the patient by positive thoughts. She should try to eliminate fear, anger, worry, anxiety and resentment from her and her patients. This requires healthy interpersonal relationships.

Develop Empathy

It will be helpful, if the nurse develops empathy with the patient. Empathy means understanding the patient's situation, feelings and motives. With proper understanding, you will be able to accept the patient as an individual.

Psychosomatic Illness

Patients with a psychosomatic illness may need more of the nurse's time, patience and attention. It is easy for the nurse to get impatient with such a patient. Such patients need help to relax and the nurse must arrange professional counselling for such patients when required.

QUESTIONS

1. Define emotion. Describe the physiological changes during emotion.
2. Define emotion and discuss emotional development in children.
3. What are emotions? Briefly mention the physiological aspects of emotions. What are their importance?
4. Write an eassay on the physiological changes in emotion.
5. Define emotion. Examine the physiological changes in emotions. What is it's importance in health and sickness? Give reference to psychosomatic aspects.
6. Write short notes on:
   a. Emotions and health
   b. Emotions
   c. Emotional problems of adolescents
7. Define emotions and feelings. How are emotions classified? What are the physical basis of emotional expressions? How is it important in health?

7 Attitudes: The Way We See Things

ATTITUDE: DEFINITION

An attitude is a predisposition to react in a persistent and characteristic manner to some situation, idea, material object or person. Our set ways of reacting to religions rituals, to our parents and teachers, to our profession or to other professions are examples of attitudes. Attitudes can be positive or negative. An attitude of respect towards elders is a positive attitude. An attitude of hatred towards a certain community, is a negative attitude.

We often remark that a certain person has a great attitude or bad attitude or should change his or her attitude. The media regularly report of topcis like drugs, smoking, marriage, dowry, divorce, sexual harassment, assisted suicides, capital punishment, fast food, etc.

An attitude is any belief or opinion that includes an evaluation of some object, person or event along a continuum from negative to positive. It predisposes us to act in a certain way toward that object, person or event.

Our attitudes have a great effect on our behaviour and have many other functions.

Attitude research has become a big business. Large amounts of money are spent each year on measuring or trying to change buyer's attitude towards consumer products and in measuring and trying to change attitude of voters towards candidates.

Components of Attitude

An attitude has three components:

a. *Cognitive* what a person knows of it and his belief about it (awareness, knowledge), how he perceives events and how he thinks about them?

b. *Affective* how he feels about it (feeling really shows concern)?
c. *Cognitive or behavioural* how he acts (psychomotor aspects) behavioural tendency both verbal and non-verbal towards the objects?

Examples

1. *Cruelty to patients:* A nurse may have definite attitudes about the way patients should be treated. Cruelty to patients may make her feel angry (affective component); because she feels strongly about it, she may be on the look out for cruelty and detect the slightest sign of any fellow nurse's impatience and irritability with a patient (cognitive component). The nurse's own behaviour could never include any act of cruelty towards any patient (behavioural component).
2. *Attitude to health:* Some people have very strong positive feeling about healthy life styles (affective componet). They will pay attention to what is said and written about healthy eating (cognitive component). One would expect such people to choose, for example, brown bread when they go shopping (behavioural component).

Factors that Determine Our Attitude

There are primarily three factors that determine our attitude. They are:

1. Environment
2. Experiences
3. Education.

Environment

Environment consists of the following:

- *Home*: Positive or negative influences
- *School*: Peer pressure
- *Work*: Supportive or over-critical supervisor
- *Media*: Television, newspapers, magazines, radio, movies
- Cultural background

- Religious background
- Traditions and beliefs
- Social environment
- Political environment.

All of these environment create a culture. Every place—be it a home, organisation or a country—has a culture.

Experiences

Our behaviour changes according to our experiences with people and events in our life. If we have a positive experience with a person, our attitude towards him becomes positive and vice versa.

Education

Knowledge strategically applied translates into wisdom, ensuring success. A teacher affects eternity. The ripple effect is immeasurable.

We are drowning in information but starving for knowledge and wisdom. Education ought to teach us not only how to make a living but also how to live.

Development of Attitudes

Our attitudes are acquired by us, and in acquiring them, we are influenced by our social, environmental, by our own thinking, our own motives, our schooling and culture norms, our early training and the factual knowledge we have about things and situations.

Heredity plays only a very small part in the development of attitudes through differences in physical characteristics and intelligence. It is mainly the environmental factors that are responsible for development of attitudes.

Early in life, a child's attitudes are shaped primarily by parents. During the period between age 12–30, the critical period, a person's attitude takes the final form. The major influences during this period are a person's peers, the information received through various media and education. After 30, attitudes change very little except that there is a tendency to become more conservative.

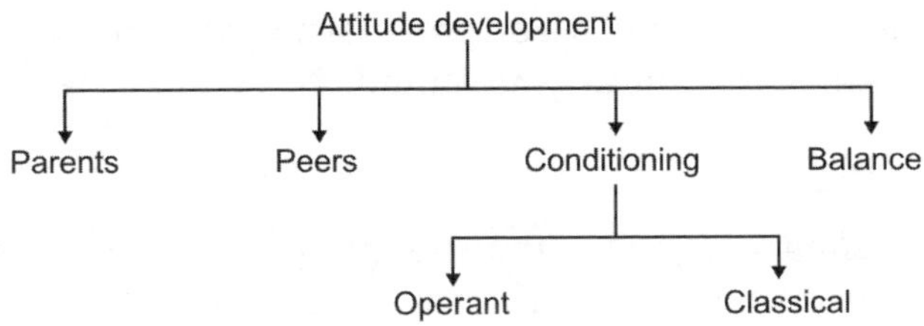

We can, however, modify the established attitudes by changing our perceptions, by controlling our motivational factors through efforts of home and school.

Family is the first place for formation of attitudes. Parents begin the information flow that forms beliefs and attitudes about things. Information provided by the parents in the earliest stages of life are very difficult to undo. Erroneous and non-adaptive attitudes moulded from parental feedback have tremendous implications for further personality development. Motives, emotions, parent-child relationships and the ways of perceiving things—all influence our attitude formation.

Attitudes originated in the family are further strengthened when they are appreciated by peers, playmates, neighbours, etc. A child is likely to internalise the attitudes of people whom he likes or whom he wishes to please. Similarly, a child tends to reject attitudes of people whom he dislikes. Attitudes accompanied by strong feelings are called sentiments.

Classical Conditioning

Griffith (1970) had people interact in small groups either in a comfortable room or one which was hot and uncomfortable. When asked to rate how much they liked the other people present in the room. Individuals in the hot room reported liking the others less than individuals in the comfortable room. In this manner, attitudes can be formed simply by association.

Instrument Conditioning

If you express an attitude to a friend, who then provides positive reinforcement by smiling or nodding, your attitude is likely to be strengthened. But if your friend provides punishment by showing or expressing disapproval, your attitude is likely to be weakened.

Balance Theory

Balance theory: It states that people prefer consistency or harmony in relationship with others. Since, balance is preferred by everyone, people develop attitudes that are harmonious with other sentimental relationships. Unbalanced structures will produce tensions and discomfort.

Measurements of Attitudes

The scientific study of attitudes requires that they be measured. In order to measure attitudes, evaluations must be translated into some number system. For some purpose, it is adequate to measure attitudes with only two categories (favourable and unfavourable). By far the most common method of measuring attitudes is the self-report method, in which people are asked to respond to questions by expressing their personal evaluations.

Public opinion (attitude) polling: Opinion polls are used either to predict something or to provide information. They are used to predict the outcome of elections, the likelihood of buying a product, or the degree of public support for implementing new policies of the Government.

POSITIVE AND NEGATIVE ATTITUDES

People with positive attitudes are caring, confident, patient and humble. Positive attitudes foster teamwork, solve problems, reduce stress and make the person an assest to his society. Negative attitudes lead to betterness, resentment, a purposeless life, ill health and high level of stress in themselves and others.

To develop a positive attitude the following suggestions will be helpful:

1. Look for the positive: Look for what is right in a person or situation instead of what is wrong.
2. Avoid procrastination: Procrastination causes fatigue and leads to a negative attitude. A completed task is fulfilling and energising.

3. Develop an attitude of gratitude: Count your blessings and not your troubles. There is a lot to be thankful for. "I complained about my bad shoes, till I met a person with no feet".

Change of attitudes: The attitudes once originated and developed in the family environment are changed by school and other world experiences. A teacher, a friend, a specific event content of school curriculum, etc. can make attitudinal changes in children.

Communication is the strongest means by which attitudinal changes can be effected in adults. Through effective communications, people can be persuaded to the extent that their attitudes may even make a shift from positive to negative. To make communication effective, three variables are to function proportionately as below:

1. The source of the communication (who says it).
2. The nature of the communication (how he says it).
3. The characteristics of the audience (to whom does he say it).

The external situation around the person also has some effect on the attitude change.

Attitudes and the nurse: The nurse who carries out an assessment of a new patient may be prevented from giving an adequate history by his attitude to his illness. The nurse who attempts to assess the patient's attitudes in order to plan appropriate care, herself brings into the situation her own complex attitude system. Her studies and her knowledge will affect her attitude to the patient's illness; her previous nursing experience influences her attitude to hospital, treatment, staff and patients.

The nurse should try to understand her patient's attitudes. Some of them enter the hospital ready and willing to cooperate, others enter hospital afraid or resentful to the ideas of receiving treatment and to the rigidity of the ward routine. Favourable or unfavourable attitudes may be the result of their own previous experience in the hospital or of the experience of their friends and relatives. These may be the result of also insufficient knowledge of what is going to happen to them when they are in the hospital.

The nurses should try to find out the causes of unfavourable attitudes and should change them into favourable ones, because favourable attitudes help in treatment and recovery. She can do this by providing better experience, by adequate explanations, by giving them a feeling of security and self-confidence, by means of efficient and skillful care, assurances and giving them a sense of being at peace by exercising patience and not being rushed. The nurse needs to develop and cultivate professional attitude which will contribute to her success in her work.

QUESTIONS

1. Define attitude. What are its components, give example?
2. How are attitudes formed?
3. How will the nurse change the negative attitude of her patient into a positive one?
4. What are the attitudes needed to become a successful nurse?

8 Habits and Skills

HABITS

Habit can be described as an automatic behaviour formed by regular repetition of an activity in more or less the same circumstances. Some of our activities like dressing, sitting or eating take place casually every day due to habits. Habits can be either good or bad.

Habit Psychology and the Nurse

Habits are time and energy saving techniques. However, difficult a task may be in the beginning, and whatever hard work it may involve, if the nurse develops a habit of doing it cheerfully and accurately, it becomes easy for her. Habits are not only mental but also physical since they require control and coordination of muscles and correct reaction time. The nursing profession requires both these.

William James (1842–1910), the founder of modern psychology in America has given the following rules for habit formation:

1. Make a strong start. It helps to have a strong need to develop a habit. A new habit will be formed more quickly if you are very strongly motivated.
2. Practise the new habit without exception until it has been firmly developed and established in your routines. If you postpone practising the habit and also allow interruptions in practice, it will be very difficult to establish a new habit.
3. Put yourself into situations which will help you develop a habit. Avoid situations that will not help. For example, if you are a late sleeper but want to develop the habit of rising early, you should try to relate with early risers and avoid late sleepers.

4. Practise a new habit until it becomes routine. Enjoy your new good habit.

The way to change bad habits in general is the same rule to form any habit as stated in James' laws above. Start with a strong desire to change; do not allow exceptions, seek support from others for your new good habit and practice the new habit. In addition, you can use problem solving techniqes to change the bad habit.

Habits build up human personality. Man should not become a slave to his habits, he should remain the master.

SKILLS

The performance of a skill is very much like that of a habit in that they are both repeated over and over again until they can be done automatically. A skill, however, is usually more complex because it involves a number of activities and makes them into a meaningful task. A motor skill is defined as the ability to perform a specialised activity effortlessly. Taking blood pressure is a skill. Brushing your teeth is a habit.

According to Munn, "a skill is a proficiency in performance of a task."

Skills help in developing and integrating one's personality. They give social prestige and status to the learner or owner and provide emotional satisfaction. When a surgeon removes a stone from the kidney of a patient or when he conducts an open heart surgery, he experiences an emotional satisfaction that arises from his skill in surgery. Skills enable an individual also to earn a living. It is the economic skill which brings prestige and status to an individual within the society.

Skills and the Nurse

Nursing is a skilled profession requiring long training period of four years. In order to develop the required skill, the nurse should follow the suggestions below:

1. Select and maintain your aim of what you want to learn.
2. Have firm determination and initiative on your part.
3. Sieze the first opportunity to act. Start on the correct track.

4. Practise the skill as a whole and not in small parts.
5. Practise often and repeat at regularly spaced intervals.
6. Evaluate and analyse what you are doing or let another person check your movements for accuracy; correct errors early.
7. *Appreciation and encouragement:* With appreciation, good act will be repeated and will help in habit formation. Learning theories by Pavlov, Skinner, Watson and others point to this fact.
8. Avoid/control all emotions and conflicts in your life.

QUESTIONS

1. Short notes on:
   - Skill and the nurse
   - Habit formation
   - Interests and their measurement.
2. (a) What are Habits?
   (b) What are the factors influencing habit formation?
   (c) How do you break bad habits?
3. (a) List the activities that you do as habit.
   (b) Illustrate James' law of habit formation by giving the steps by which you formed habits.

9 The Learning Process

One of the most important characteristics of human being is their capacity to learn. Our personality—our habits, skills, knowledge, attitudes, interests and character is largely the result of learning.

DEFINITION

Learning has been defined as a permanent change in behaviour that occurs as a result of practice or experience.

A little girl, being indisposed is taken to a hospital. The nurse prepares the syringe which the little girl watches with interest. The nurse injects the medicine and the girl feels pain. When the little girl is taken to the nurse next time, she starts screaming when the nurse takes the syringe. She had learned by experience that injections are painful. Learning caused changes in her behaviour.

Learning is central to all our behaviour as we learn to speak, write, think and perceive. Our attitudes and emotional expressions are also learned behaviours. There are three important factors in the definition of learning:

1. Learning brings change in behaviour (usually for the better).
2. Change takes place through practice or experience and not due to maturation.
3. The change in behaviour should be relatively permanent lasting for years, months or weeks.

Conditions Affecting Learning

1. *Intelligence* or mental faculty which involves the activity of the sensory adjustment and motor mechanisms of the body. Intelligence is related to heredity, nutrition and IQ. Children with low IQ are poor learners or may not learn at all.

2. *Motivation*
3. *Age:* The capacity to learn improves upto 23 or 24 years of age. After 40, it declines.
4. *Learning situation:* Physical facilities for learning namely institutions, teachers, textbooks, audiovisual aids promote learning.
5. *Physical health* deaf, blind, dumb, chronically ill persons (handicapped) cause difficulty to learn.
6. *Mental health* Worries, anxieties and fears interfere with learning.

Types of Learning

1. Cognitive learning (knowledge)
2. Affective learning (attitudes)
3. Psychomotor learning (skills).

MODES, METHODS OR THEORIES OF LEARNING

1. Trial and error
2. Theory of conditioned reflexes
   a. Classical conditioning
   b. Operant conditioning
3. Cognitive learning
   a. Insight learning
   b. Sign learning.

Trial and Error Method

Edward Lee Thorndike (1874–1949), the American psychologist, considered as the father of educational psychology, conducted a series of experiments (1911) on trial and error method of learning by animals.

Experiment

A hungry rat was set free at the entrance of a wooden maze which contained many pathways from the entrance to the centre. But all the ways except one were blocked somewhere in the middle. A piece of bread was placed in the centre of the maze. Seeing the bread, the hungry rat rushed to get it. It happened to enter the wrong path which was obstructed in the middle. Consequently it had to return to the entrance but only to try other paths till it reached the bread. The next day, it made less errors. The experiment continued for several days till the rat was able to identify the right path at the very first glance without trying out other paths. Thorndike conducted similar experiments on a number of animals, e.g. monkeys, dogs, hens and cats. The errors were reduced as the trials were repeated. Stimulus-Response, i.e. SR connections were made.

From the cat's experiment and several other similar experiments, Thorndike formulated certain laws of learning. According to Thorndike all learning is trial and error.

Laws of Effective Learning

1. *Law of effect:* Any response followed by a reward (food) will be strengthened. Any response which is unsuccessful will be weakened.
2. *Law of exercise:* The law of exercise states that there is a direct relationship between repetition and the strength of the stimulus-response bond. The law of exercise is based on the law of use and law of disuse. As per the law of use, any task that is repeated shows a tendency for the strengthening of the bond and as per the law of disuse any task that is not repeated shows a tendency for the weakening of the bond. The learned activity (reading, writing, typing, singing, drawing, dancing, etc.) is learned by constant practice over a long period.
3. *Law of readiness:* Learning takes place best when a person is ready to learn. If a person is ready to act, acting gives him satisfaction. A person cannot learn if he is not ready to learn. Readiness includes motivation, inclination, attitude or mindset.

Thorndike ignored the role of intelligence and insight in learning. Many scientific discoveries have taken place suddenly without any prior trial and error. Quite often individuals learn suddenly by insight rather than by trial and error which is a very time consuming process.

Learning by Trial and Error

The method of trial and error is used when:

a. The learner is completely motivated and sees the goal clearly. The rat tries to get into the centre of the maze only because it is hungry and sees that there is food at the centre of the maze.
b. When perception or learned activities alone are not sufficient.
c. When the learner fails to find the solution to the problem through perception, understanding, intelligence and language. Then he proceeds blindly, tries in various directions, commits errors; eliminates them and finally arrives at the correct response.

Classical Conditioning

The study of classical conditioning began in the early years of 20th century when Ivan Pavlov, a Russian physiologist who had already won the Nobel prize (1904) for research on digestion, turned his attention to learning. While studying digestion Pavlov, noticed that a dog began to salivate at the mere sight of the food dish. Pavlov decided to see whether a dog could be taught to associate food with other things, such as a light or a bell.

Pavlov's Experiments

In Pavlov's experiments, a researcher first attached a capsule to a dog's salivary gland to measure salivary flow. A bell was rung, every time, the dog was given the meat powder. This was repeated several times. Later Pavlov observed that the dog salivated at the mere sound of the bell, followed by the meat powder. Thus, the dog had been conditioned to respond to a new stimulus which was previously an unconditioned response.

The meat powder is the unconditioned stimulus (UCS); salivation is the unconditioned response (UCR) Sound of the bell is the conditioned stimulus (CS) and salivation at the sound of the bell is the conditioned response (CR).

Pavlov's theory is that CS (bell) simply as a result of pairing with the UCS (meat powder) acquires the capacity to substitute the UCS in evoking the response. This means that an association is formed between the CS and the UCS, so that CS becomes the equivalent of the UCS in eliciting response.

Pavlov believed that this association took place in the brain. Two areas of the brain, one for the UCS and the other for the CS became activated during classical conditioning and the activation of UCS area resulted in a reflex or automatic response.

Extinction and Spontaneous Recovery

When a CS is presented alone without the UCS for a number of trials, the strength of the CS gradually decreases and this process is called extinction. Thus, when the bell is presented alone without the meat powder for a number of trials, salivation gradually decreases. After a response has been extinguished, it recovers some of its strength with the passage of time. This is known as spontaneous recovery. This implies that the extinction procedure while decreasing the strength of a conditioned response does not entirely remove the tendency to respond to CS. Reconditioning is more rapid than original conditioning. Reconditioning occurs when CS and UCS from original conditions are paired again.

Generalisation

Stimulus generalisation is the tendency to give conditioned response to stimuli that are similar in some way to the conditioned stimulus but have never been paired with the unconditioned stimulus. The greater the similarly of these stimuli to the original conditioned stimulus, the greater is the amount of generalisation.

Stimulus generalisations are responsible for developing phobias in people. A child who is attacked by a dog can develop a fear for furred animals and even for Santa Claus who has a white beard. These irrational fears can be eliminated by the principle of extinction.

Descrimination

This is a process that is complimentary to generalisation. It occurs when the individual learns to distinguish between similar stimuli and to respond differently to each. While generalisation occurs due to similarities, discrimination results due to differences. Selective reinforcement and extinction cause descrimination. For example, in an experiment with animals, lights S1 and S2 on adjacent windows served as conditioned stimuli which lead to conditioned blinking to that light which was followed by an air puff to the eye as a conditioned stimulus. On the first day only S1 was presented and reinforced. By generalisation it was developed for S2 also.

When on the second day trials with S1 and S2 intermingled and presented when only S1 was reinforced, conditioned blinking occurred only for S1. This shows that the animal has discriminated between S1 and S2. Discrimination is the opposite of generalisation.

Processes like extinction, spontaneous recovery, generalisation and discrimination are being successfully used in behaviour therapy. Many of the unpleasant emotional responses that are the causative factors for many abnormal behaviours can be eliminated by using the principles of classical conditioning.

Learning by Classical Conditioning

The principles of classical conditioning can be used in the following areas of animal and human learning:

1. *Developing good habits:* Good habits such as cleanliness, respect for elders, and punctuality, etc. can be brought about by using principles of classical conditioning.
2. *Breaking of bad habits and elimination of conditioned fears:* All learning is acquired in the social environment.
3. *Training of animals:* Animal trainers have been using the principle of classical conditioning for long without being much aware of the underlying mechanism.
4. *Use in psychotherapy:* In deconditioning emotional fears in mental patients.
5. To develop favourable or unfavourable attitude towards learning, teacher and the school.

Anxiety which is a common symptom of emotional disorder is a fear that is induced through classical conditioning. For example, a person develops fear of automobiles because of his painful experience of an accident.

JB Watson, father of the behaviourist school, showed that it is possible to condition children in the same way as dogs. He conditioned his nine months old child Albert to become afraid of furry animals by frightening him with a loud noise, every time he played with a previously beloved furry toy.

A number of activities, we perform in our day-to-day life are merely conditioned reflexes learned through the process of conditioning. Some psychiatric symptoms may be the result of conditioning. Fear of open undefined spaces, of sharp objects, of blood, of carrying out certain treatments may have occurred as a result of conditioning without the person's knowledge.

Operant Conditioning or Instrumental Conditioning

Instrumental conditioning is associated with the works of EL Thorndike and BF Skinner. Thorndike was the first to conduct laboratory experiments (1898) on operant conditioning leading to the formulation of the law of effect which formed the basis of the principle of reinforcement. But it was Skinner who made operant conditioning popular with experiments on pigeons, rats and human beings.

Skinner placed a rat inside a glass box (Skinner box) containing a lever and food tray. The animal was free to explore the box. Whenever, the lever in the box was pressed, automatically a pellet of food was dropped on the tray. By a mechanical device the number of times the rat pressed on the lever was recorded. Pressing of the lever was the response to be learned (the operant response) and the food was the stimulus consequence (reinforcement). The rate of presses increased notably with the rewarding of the rat with food each time he pressed the bar. By reinforcement the rat learned the instrumental response. Reinforcement can be either positive (rewards) or negative (punishment).

Operants are actions which animals and human beings do like walking, smiling, watching televisions, etc. The learner has to "operate" on his environment. The term "instrumental" points to the fact that the learner has some control over his circumstances. His action is instrumental to what happens to him. Instrumental conditioning involves more activity on the part of the learner than classical conditioning. Generally, behaviour directed towards gaining a reward or avoiding a punishment are examples of instrumental action. Intention and achievement are important in this kind of learning.

Types of Instrumental Conditioning

By this method, it is possible to teach an individual to make a particular response or withhold it by providing him either reward or punishment. Positive reinforcement is used in reward training. For example, giving an individual his due allowance when he makes the desired response. When rewards are used to withhold a response that is not desired, it is called omission training. For example, if a child is offered a candy for giving up nail biting. Escape training refers to the use of negative reinforcement to increase the frequency of a desired response. Telling a convict that good conduct on his part will secure him remission of sentence is an example for escape training. Punishment training is used to make the learner stop performing an undesired response. For example, scolding a child for using impolite language.

Shaping

Shaping refers to the reinforcing of closer approximation for performing a desired response. This consists of learning graduated steps, when each following step has a resemblance to the desired performance and it is known as the method of successive approximations. For example, in language teaching, the child may at the beginning say "Maaa" ——— Mrrrr ——— Maar ——— and finally "Mother".

Behaviour Modification

Operant conditioning is used in a form of treatment known as behaviour modification. Patients with behaviour disorders have successfully learnt to use socially acceptable behaviour within a relatively short time. Mentally retarded children have learnt self-help skills such as use of toilet 'and dressing and undressing previously considered too difficult.

Comparison between classical and operant conditioning	
Classical conditioning	**Operant conditioning**
Response is elicited	Response is emitted or not, the UCS will be presented
Time interval between CS and the UCS is rigidly fixed	Time interval depends on the organism's own behaviour
The unconditioned stimulus (UCS) occurs without regard to the subject's behaviour	The reward is contingent upon the occurrence of response
Association between stimulus-response (S-R) is on the basis of law of contiguity (things occurring closer in time and space get associated)	Association between stimulus-response (S-R) is on the basis of law of effect (effect of reward and punishment)
There is pairing of UCS and CS	No pairing of UCS and CS but pairing of a response and the reinforcing stimulus which follows
Reinforcement comes first as food is presented first to elicit the response	Reinforcement is provided after the response is made by the organism
Unconditioned stimulus (UCS) is presented regardless of whether the conditioned response (CR) occurs	Stimulus is presented only if the organism makes the desired response
Stimulus oriented	Response oriented
Essence of learning is stimulus substitution	The essence of learning is response modification
Involuntary response	Voluntary response
Involves autonomic nervous system	Involves central nervous system
Organism is passive	Organism is active
Underlines our learning of physiological and emotional reactions. Learned reflexes are acquired this way.	Underlines our acquisition of habits and skills

There are many techniques which can be used and their application to specific patients has to be so carefully planned that many colleges of nursing now offer post basic courses in behaviour therapy. For behaviour modification, one must analyse how complex the desired behaviour is. To eat with a spoon, for example, has many subskills, such as sitting down, putting the hands on the table and not into the soup, holding the spoon by the handle and lifting the spoon in the correct direction. Any one of these activities can be separately rewarded without waiting until a whole plateful of soup has been eaten. This is known as 'behaviour shaping.'

While nurses should know what reward pleases a patient most, she must also learn to ignore inappropriate responses of her patients. A systematic attempt to decondition by making new associations with pleasure stimuli is being done in psychotherapy. Patients have been helped by this method to overcome disabling fears of open spaces, sharp objects and other phobias. Alcoholism and sexual deviation have been successfully treated by the reverse process, of establishing a conditioned link between nausea and drinking or sexually deviant behaviour.

Principle of instrument conditioning is used in programmed learning and in personalised system of instruction (PSI).

Cognitive Theories of Learning

In more complex forms of learning, perception and knowledge or cognition processes play the vital role. According to cognitive theorists, learning cannot be explained in terms of S-R (stimulus-response) association alone. They propose that a learner forms a cognitive structure in memory which organises information into relationships and meanings without any known reinforcement. New associations are formed and new relationships are perceived along events, simply as a result of having experienced these events. Links are made among stimuli, so that stimulus-stimulus (S-S) associations are learned.

Learning by Insight (Gestalt)

Thorndike ignored the role of intelligence and insight learning. Many scientific discoveries have taken place suddenly without any prior trial and error. Quite often individuals learn suddenly by insight rather than by trial and error, which is a very time consuming process.

Learning by Insight Theory

It was developed by a group of Gestalt psychologists, Kurt Koffka, Wolfgang Kohler and Max Wertheimer who concluded that the individual learns by his ability known as insight and not by blind trial and error. According to them, a person can deduce the solution by insight if he perceives the situation as a whole. The situation viewed as a whole will definitely look different from that viewed through its parts. The whole of an object or situation is not merely the sum total of its parts like water is quite different from its elements hydrogen and oxygen. Sum total of the parts may create a new entity which is called as Gestalt. The emergence of a Gestalt, produces in an individual an insight into the problem.

The most famous experiments conducted by Kohler in relation to insight were those conducted with a chimpanzee called Sultan. Some bananas were hung inside the cage of hungry Sultan who was then given two sticks so constructed that they could be fitted together.

The hungry Sultan tried to get the bananas by extending out his hands. Then he took up one of the sticks and tried to pull the bananas, an effort which he kept up for one hour. Then he got tired and started to play with the sticks. Meanwhile, one end of one stick got incidentally fastened into the ring fixed on the end of other stick with the result that both the sticks were joined together. Now Sultan used this joined stick to pull in the bananas and succeeded.

The Gestalt psychologists made a number of such experiments and concluded that individuals learn by insight which emerges suddenly as a result of perceiving the situation as a whole. Sultan's sudden learning was due to insight developed from his perception of the total situation consisting of the cage, sticks and bananas as a whole.

Characteristics of Learning by Insight

1. Insight is sudden.
2. Insight is due to understanding.
3. Insight alters perception.
4. Old objects appear in new patterns and organisation due to insight.
5. Higher species of animals including man has more insight than members of lower species.
6. Insight develops usually after some trial and error.

While classical conditioning and operant conditioning (trial and error) belong to the stimulus-response (S-R) theories of learning, insight learning belongs to the cognitive learning stimulus stimulus (S-S) theories.

Insight is often used in problem solving puzzles and riddles. To emphasize the suddenness of the solution, it is also called as "Aha experience".

Steps in Learning Process

1. Motivation within the learner.
2. Goal or goals become related to the motivation.
3. Barriers of difficulties are perceived and experienced and tension rises. Strong barriers may cause excessive tension which may altogether discourage and confuse the learner.
4. The search for an appropriate solution to the problem or an appropriate line of action to reach his goal.
5. The most appropriate line of action is selected and practised; inappropriate behaviours dropped.

Factors Influencing Learning

Learning depends upon three main factors:
1. Nature of the learner.
2. Nature of the learning material or task to be learned.
3. Nature of the learning situation or learning methods.

Nature of the Learner

a. *Perception:* Sense organs are the gateways of knowledge. The process of perception and the factors related to perception should be perfect.
b. *Organic defects:* Visual defects like hyperopia, myopia astigmatism and colour blindness can affect learning adversely. Similar is the case with hearing impairment and infections.
c. *Fatigue:* Both mental and physiological; compulsive learning, loneliness, strain, restlessness and boredom can cause mental

fatigue. Studying in a room lacking fresh air and sunlight and in places where waste materials and toxic substances are acumulated can cause physiological fatigue.

d. *Time of the day:* There is no variation in efficiency of learning throughout the day, provided other factors are present. Even adverse environmental conditions like heat and noise can be overcome with learner's willpower.
e. *Age and learning:* The capacity to learn improves up to 23 or 24 years. After 40 it declines.

Nature of Learning Materials

Less the number of learning elements in a material and less complexity, easier the learning. Meaningful learning is easier than learning a material without knowing the meaning not learning. The better the individual elements of learning material be distinguished, the faster they are learned.

Nature of the Learning Method (Making Learning more Effective)

a. *Definite goal*: With a clear goal in mind, the student works towards a definite purpose. Clear aim enhances motivation. Intention to learn ensures better learning.
b. *Knowledge of results or psychological feedback:* Frequent and regular review of the amount of progress being made towards the goal, acts as a strong motive to promote continuing effort on the part of the learner.
c. *Distribution of practice periods:* Shorter practice periods are more effective than longer periods and when distributed over several days yields better result. This will reduce mental fatigue.
d. *Whole versus part method:* This is as per Gestalt theory. With easy units whole method should be adopted. If the material is difficult, smaller units can be learnt but they should still be as large wholes as a learner can manage efficiently. Try to learn in natural units. Rhyming helps to learn poems.
e. *Logical learning:* Instead of rote memorisation you should try to grasp the meaning of the text. Logical learning calls for an arrangement and also assimilation with ideas in mind.

f. *Rest:* Take rest in between your studies as mental fatigue prolongs the study process.
g. *Level of anxiety:* Mild degree of anxiety can be a useful aid to learning but undue worry, anxiety and nervousness will have an inhibiting and interfering effect.
h. Overlearning/repetitions at regular intervals help to retain the material over a longer period of time.

Learning curves: The rate of learning can be quantitatively measured by plotting it on a graph. In some cases, we find that the increase in learning is small in the beginning but the rate increases with the progress of learning. This is called positively, accelerated curve (Fig. 9.1). In such a curve, an increasing rate is shown throughout. If the gains in the beginning are relatively more and decrease as learning progresses we get a negatively accelerated curve. Negative acceleration is characterised by initial increase in gains followed by decrease with practice. These curves may be obtained for tasks which are not able to sustain the motivation of a student. Positively-accelerated curves are obtained when learning of simple things are involved.

A learning curve for tasks of uniform difficulty shows a slow start followed by increase in learning, then decrease followed by a period of almost no learning and then a period of learning or reaching the limit (S-shaped curve) the stages are referred to as initial lag, increasing gain, decreasing gain, plateau and spurt.

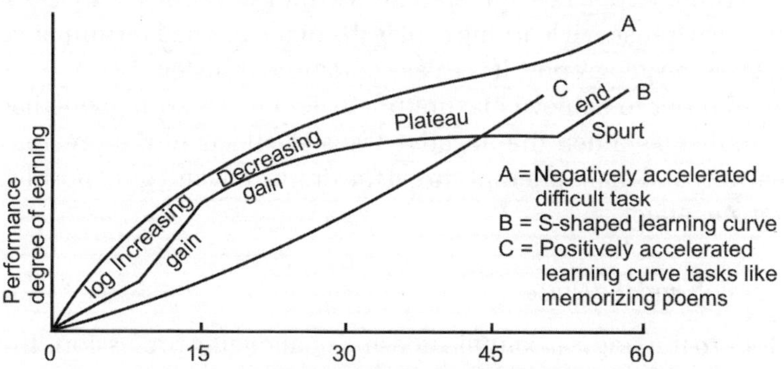

Fig. 9.1: Learning curves

Transfer of Learning

Transfer of learning or training occurs when learning of one set of material influences the learning of another set of material later. For example, driving a new car. The movements and responses in driving a new car will have similarities and differences when compared to movements and responses in driving the old car. The individual has to adapt his old habits and learn new ones.

To demonstrate the effects of transfer of learning, the following experiment is useful. Two groups of subjects are used. The first, experimetnal group learns task A and then task B. The second group (the control group) learns task (B) only without learning task (A). If the experimental group learns task (B) more easily and effectively than the control group, we say that positive transfer has taken place. Positive transfer means the learning of the earlier task (A) has facilitated the learning of the later task (B). On the other hand, if the experimental group is found to be more difficult in learning task B, with poor performance, we may say that negative transfer has occurred. Negative transfer means that the learning of the earlier task (A) has interfered with or hindered the learning of the later task (B). If both the experimental and control groups learn the latter task (B) in an equal manner, no transfer or neutral transfer has occurred.

For example, if learning to play the piano has facilitated the learning to play the violin, it is a case of positive transfer of learning. If learning Telugu has hindered the learning of Tamil, it is a case of negative transfer. If learning to play the piano has had no influence in learning geography, it is a case of neutral transfer.

In order to achieve maximum efficiency of learning, one has to reduce as much the negative transfer effects of the previous learning and make attempts to get maximum advantage of positive transfer effect.

Learning and the Nurse

Modern nursing is a complicated and challenging profession. The student nurse must have a clear goal and interest to learn. She has to acquire a lot of information from books, lectures and discussion.

There are many complicated skills she has to learn with repeated practice.

Everyday newer techniques are being introduced in medical science. The knowledge of learning process is helpful to the nurse not only while she is a student but throughout her career. The more she is prepared to receive new ideas, make new adjustments and learn new techniques, the more she will be successful in her profession.

Every patient admitted in the hospital, has something unique about him. The nurse should have good understanding and learn more about each patient. This will lead to better adjustment and early cure.

Some diseases leave the patient crippled in one way or another. The nurse has to teach him new ways and techniques to substitute for the function of the crippled organ. This requires knowledge of the learning process by the patient and the nurse.

QUESTIONS

1. Define learning. Discuss the nature and steps in learning.
2. Illustrate Pavlov's classical conditioning with laboratory experiment.
3. State laws of learning and factors which affect effective learning.
4. Briefly outline the special features of classical conditioning and operant conditioning.
5. What is learning? Bring out the differences between classical and operant learning.
6. Define learning. Discuss different methods of learning. Give examples of the instrumental learning. How is it used in habit formation?
7. Short notes on:
   a. Individual differences in learning
   b. Learning
   c. Learning types
   d. Learning by insight.

10 Remembering and Forgetting

Memory was one of the first phenomena to be studied in a psychological laboratory (Ebbinghaus, 1864). Without memory there would be no learning. We would react to each occurrence of a situation as though it had not yet been experienced. The power to store experiences and to bring them into the field of consciousness sometime after the experience has occurred is called memory. The current trend in the study of memory emphasises *cognitive or mental process*. Cognition concerns the internal processing of information received from the senses. One aspect of this processing is memory. Memory is the encoding, storage and retrieval of information.

Memory System—Information Processing

Ideas about memory that emphasize the processing of information in stages or steps are known as information processing theories. According to psychologist, John Kihlstron, university of Arisona, this approach is modelled after high speed computer (1987).

The memorising process are organised in the form of memory traces which functions like a computer.

Memory is said to consist of three cognitive processes mentioned in its definition—encoding, storage and retrieval.

Encoding is the process of receiving sensory input and transforming it into a code that can be stored.

Storage is the process of actually putting the coded information into memory.

Retrieval is the process of gaining access to the encoded, stored information when it is to be used.

Types of Memory

Depending upon the difference in the rates of decay of the information, mainly three kinds of storage are described. They are:

1. Sensory memory (SM) or immediate memory
2. Short-term memory (STM) or working memory and
3. Long-term memory (LTM).

Sensory Memory or Immediate Memory

Sensory memory stores incoming information in a sensory register which has large capacity. Information in sensory register lasts for a very short duration ranging from fraction of a second to a few seconds. Sensory image is like the flash of letters on a screen or the auditory image of a spoken word. The materials of sensory memory may be processed into short-term or long-term memory or they may be discarded.

Short-term Memory (STM) or Working Memory

Short-term memory holds a relatively small amount of information, about seven items or chunks, for a short period of 15–30 seconds. The type of information stored consists of sounds, images, words or sentences. Information is lost from STM by being displaced by new inputs. Information from STM may be transferred to LTM through either maintenance or elaborate rehearsal (Fig. 10.1).

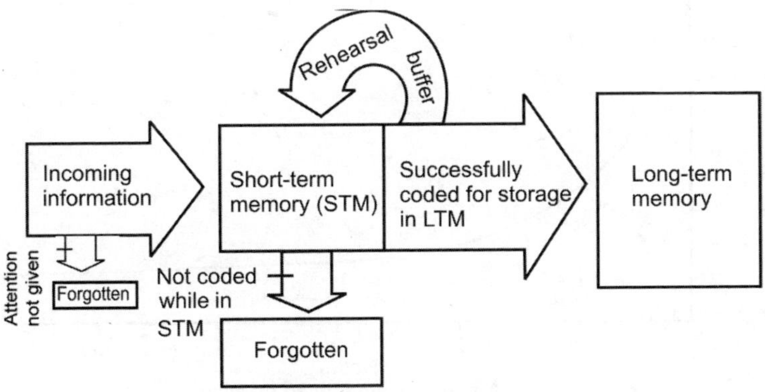

Fig. 10.1: STM and LTM

Long-term Memory (LTM)

LTM has the unlimited capacity to store information for days, months, years and even a life time. Information may be lost, or at least not retrieved, from long-term memory because of difficulties in the search process or because of interference by other long-term memories.

It is by LTM that you always remember your name, your father's name, date of birth and other personal data (Fig. 10.2).

FORGETTING

Munn (1967) defines forgetting as the loss, permanent or temporary, of the ability to recall or recognise something learned earlier. Sometimes what we think is forgotten in real sense is not forgotten because it has never been encoded and stored in the first place. Many students complain that they do not remember the contents after attending the class or forget after reading the text.

This is due to lack of attention. Some information does not reach STM from sensory register or due to inadequate encoding and rehersal, the information may not have been transferred from STM to LTM.

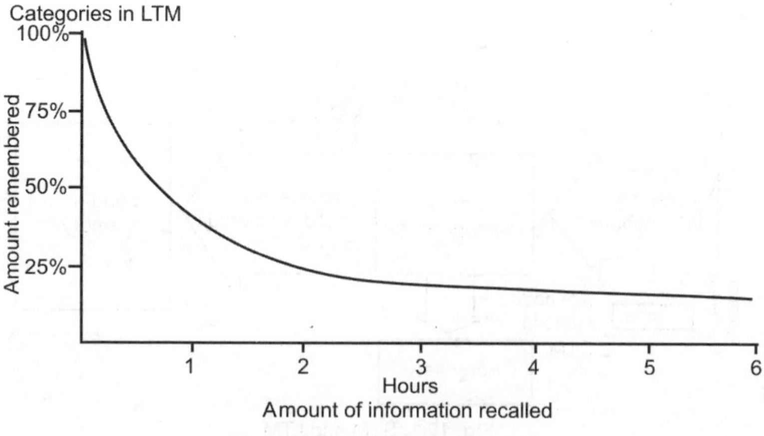

Fig. 10.2: Curve of forgetting

Causes of Forgetting

Faulty Memory Process

Many times we forget as memory does not match events which had occurred. This happens due to the constructive processes, i.e. certain materials may be simplified or changed during encoding. We remember the gist or meaning of what we have read or heard, but not the actual words themselves.

Interference

Learning new things interfere with memory of what is learned earlier and prior learning interferes with memory of things learned later.

a. *Retroactive inhibition:* This is a technical name of new learning interfering with material previously learned. This is a backward effect. An experimental design for the retroactive inhibition is given in Table 10.1.

   For example, you may learn one chapter of physiology in activity I, then learn one chapter of Anatomy in activity II, then try to recall what you have learned in physiology. The amount of information you forgot would be due to rectroactive inhibition caused by learning anatomy.

   The control group learns the same chapter of physiology, rest for sometime, and afterwards find the recall much better as there is no retroactive inhibition.

b. *Proactive inhibition:* When prior learning interferes with the learning and recall of a new material, it is proactive inhibition. This is a forward process.

Table 10.1: Retroactive inhibition

Groups		Activity	
	I	II	III (Test)
Experimental	Learn A	Learn B	Recall A
Control	Learn A	Rest or unrelated activity	Recall A

Table 10.2: Proactive inhibition

Groups		Activity	
	I	II	III (Test)
Experimental	Learn A	Learn B	Recall B
Control	Rest or unrelated activity	Learn B	Recall B

An experimental design for the proactive inhibition is given in Table 10.2.

Suppose you learn English (A), then French (B) you would find that the study of English interfering with your recall of French due to proactive inhibition, i.e. interference with subsequent memory.

In both types of interference, it has been found that the effect of interference is less with meaningful material and after attaining some mastery in the subject. Time tabling of lessons in various educational settings is designed to reduce forgetting due to interference. Very dissimilar subjects follow each other. For example, in schools, a language might follow mathematics, in colleges of nursing, practical nursing then anatomy. At the beginning of your course you should try to allot different study times to similar subjects to avoid interference.

Other Types of Interference

Forgetting occurs owing to several other types of interference like items in the STM interfere with each other thus are continually forgotten. One tends to remember items at the start of a list (primary effect) and at the end of a list (recency effect) better than items in the middle (serial position effect).

Items in the LTM interact with each other, old items can be distorted or changed by the new inputs.

Some inputs are rejected by the lower centres of the brain because they are meaningless or unimportant while other inputs are deliberately repressed.

Encoding, Organisation and Retrieval Problems

If the stored information is not encoded well or organised at the time of learning, it is forgotten. Retrieval cues are important in memory as we may not be able to recall an information in one situation but may spontaneously remember in another situation. Retrieval is facilitated by organisation of the stored material and the presence of retrieval cues that can guide our search through LTM for stored information. In the absence of proper retrieval cues, the desired items stored with LTM will not be found. Sometimes, you cannot recall something while actively searching for it but after giving up that search, while doing something else, you recall that information. This is because your new activity has generated new retrieval cues.

Motivated Forgetting

Many lapses of memory in daily life are due to motivated forgetting. We may forget the names of people whom we hate. We forget to buy a particular edible item, which the housewife had asked to buy, probably because it is not to our liking. Repression theory holds that we forget because the retrieval of memories would be painful or unacceptable in some way.

Visitors to patients sometimes indulge in recollections of all the sad and unfortunate experiences which they remember suddenly when the association with hospital. Sickness and death bring those memories to the fore. Patients do not find stories of other people's suffering, operations, treatments and misfortunes at all comforting. Nurses may have to help visitors to remember positive, encouraging and hopeful types of conversation by their own cheerful, optimistic attitude to visitors.

The patient may appear to forget his family and his work and may remember only the events which occur in the hospital. His conversation is about the wards, the nurses, other patients. He appears to have forgotten his family. Children in hospital show this to a very marked degree.

Emotional factors also play an important role in forgetting. If we encode while is one emotional state and try to recall it while in another, our recall suffers.

Anxiety or guilt producing material are more often forgotten than pleasant experiences. Suppose in a particular class, you were scolded by the instructor. You are likely to forget most of what was taught in that class that day. This is why punishment is not, in the long run, effective in promoting learning.

Psychologists have also found that some persons cannot forget unpleasant experiences easily and this is related to personality.

Amnesia-Forgetting during Sickness

Amnesia refers to loss of memory due to disease. The person may forget his past experiences or may have impaired ability to encode, store and to retrieve making new memory difficult. Amnesia is a profound memory deficit due to either the loss of what has been stored or to the inability to form new memories.

Amnesias are classified into two types: Biological and psychological.

a. *Biological amnesias:* These are caused by brain malfunctions. Examples are transient global amnesia, alcohol induced amnesia and the amnesia caused by certain diseases of the brain. Transient global amnesia is a shortlived amnesia attack characterized by retrograde and anterograde amnesia. High doses of alcohol result in amnesia for the events that occurred while drunk. In addition, heavy drinking over a period of years can produce brain damage and a pattern of systems known as the Korsakoff syndrome. Anterograde amnesia and some loss of remote memory characterize the memory problems of this syndrome. Senile dementia and primary degenerative dementia, of which Alzheimer's disease is an example are instances of brain diseases that have amnesia as a major symptom.
b. *Psychological amnesia:*
   i. *Childhood amnesia:* It is due to the differences in the ways young children and older people encode and store information. As adults, much of our memory is encoded verbally and tied into networks or schemata that are language based. But the young child without language encodes memories in a non-verbal form, perhaps storing information as images or feelings. Early childhood

memories are thus said to be stored in forms no longer available to us as verbal adults. Our language dominated memories do not have retrieval cues appropriate for gaining access to the image and feeling memories of early childhood.

Perhaps the memory machine is just not able to store long-term memories until its maturation is essentially finished. Language ability and memory develop together because both depends on brain maturation. Repression is another explanation given for childhood and dream amnesias.

ii. *Dream amnesia:* In dream amnesia, the difference between the symbol system in dreams and in waking makes the waking retrieval of any information encoded during dreaming difficult.

While usually considered to be psychological, childhood and dream amnesia have a biological basis—the immaturity of the brain in childhood amnesia and the difference between the brain states in dreaming and in waking for dream amnesia. The forgetting of defensive amnesia protects the amnesiac from the guilt or anxiety that can accompancy intense, intolerable life situations and conflicts.

Memory and Brain Damage

When the brain is damaged by accident, operation, drugs or toxins, remembering is impaired. The amount of forgetting is related to the extent of brain damage. Because forgetting takes place most rapidly immediately after learning, before consolidation has taken place and much more slowly later on, the material most recently learnt is most completely forgotten after head injury. Old knowledge remains intact.

Patients, who suffer from concussion may have forgotten what they were doing at the time of the accident. On recovery from electroconvulsive therapy, epilepsy fits or an anaesthetic, the patient may forget where he placed his belongings, what was the last meal he ate or which part of the ward he was in.

METHODS TO IMPROVE MEMORY

Proper Learning Method

With proper learning method with training, practice and motivation, memory can be improved. Learning by whole rather than by parts, improves learning. Similarly recitation method helps to memorise better than continued re-reading of the same material.

Our recall process can be improved by keeping ourselves away from harmful emotional factors, building self-confidence and making the right associations. Learner's will, his interest, span of attention and the right learning methods have vital roles to play in the process of remembering. Memory training aims to achieve a good memory (Fig. 10.3).

Mnemonics or Memory Tricks

Mnemonics, comes from the Greek word for memory and refers to the specific memory improvement techniques. Most mnemonics techniques rely on the linking or association of to-be-remembered material with a systematic and organised set of images or words

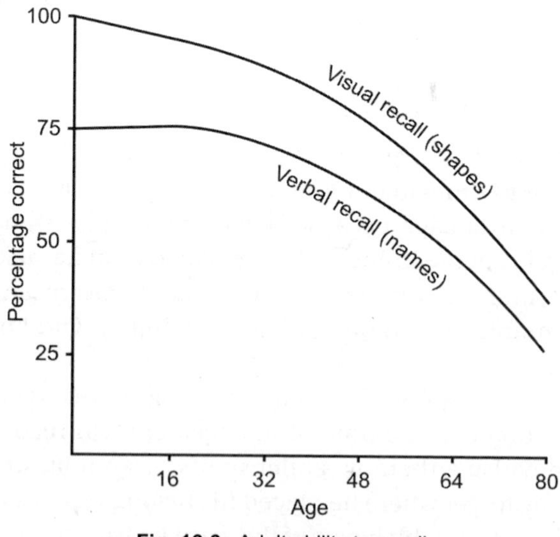

Fig. 10.3: Adult ability to recall

with which we are very familiar, and therefore can provide reminder cues.

Memory Pegs

Memory pegs with the analogy of a clockroom in mind, the reminder cues are called memory pegs to hang the to-be-remembered items, e.g. the letters of the word VIBGYOR can be used as "pegs" on which to hang the names of rainbow colours-violet, indigo, blue, green, yellow, orange and red.

The Method of Loci

The word loci means "places". The memory pegs of this system are parts of your image of a scene. The scene can be a street, a building with roads the layout of a college campus, a kitchen or anything that can be visualized clearly and contains a number of discrete items in specific locations to serve as memory pegs. Supposing you want to remember for examination, classical conditioning. Then start by imagining a dog, experimental room, food, bell and any person as an experimenter. Reherse this image over and over until it is well established in your mind. After you have formed your image, associate the events like stimulus substitution and extinction with this. The trick is to make association with as many concepts as needed.

Rhyming System

Think of the words that rhyme with numbers 1 is a bun, 2 is shoe, 3 is a tree, 4 is a door and so on. Now when you have a list to remember, you can associate the items on the list with your images of the numbers. If the first item on a grocery list is coffee imagine a steamed cup of coffee next to a plate of buns; if the second item is hamburger, you might see a giant shoe squashing hamburger into a patty and so on.

Make a Story

If you have a list of unrelated items to remember a useful memory devise is to relate the items in a made-up story.

The story starts with the first item on the list and each succeeding items is included in that order. Doing this gives coherence and meaning to the otherwise unrelated items. It is a form of elaborative encoding.

Chunking

Suppose you want to remember your credit card number -201416099001, you can break the numbers into chunks, the first four digits could be remembered as the year you passed your school or associate with any significant thing that happened in that year—next four digits could also be taken as date, e.g. some one's birthday. The last four numbers form a chunk that is easy to remember by itself.

Overlearning

Retention is greater when subject matter is well-learned. Over-learning is the term used to describe practice that continues after a perfect recall has been scored.

Studying to Remember

Here are some tips to improve your memory:

a. Study is work and takes time, so plan *a study time table* to cover the study content. Stick to this schedule firmly. If you study hard during your scheduled time, you will have plenty of time for your friends and television.
b. Rehersal is crucial for transfering information from STM to LTM. Maintenance rehersal consists of merely repeating information while elaborative rehersal consists of thinking about what is rehersed in an effort to relate it to other things that you know or are learning. You should spend half of your study time in elaborative rehearsal.

   Make notes of important points as all the details of information cannot be remembered. Revise these notes often. You use imagery to visualize the material you are learning and give auditory stimulation by reading aloud. For example, while studying nervous system, visualize the structure of nervous system with minute detail and also read loudly. Multichannel stimulation will improve your memory.

c. Remember the importance of *organization*. Textbooks like this one, are organized by headings, to provide a kind of outline. As you reherse elaborately, give your own organisation, under different topic headings and provide your own retrieval cues. For visual images of abstract ideas make a map of the contents in your mind.
d. Give a feedback to yourselves by testing your grasp. Do some additional work on any weak spots. Revise the areas where you could not remember. By testing yourself, you will be practising your retrieving skills.
e. Review before examination. Try to overlearn but do not get anxious as you have seen high anxiety level would interfere with your remembering.
f. Give some short rest pauses between your study time. It would help to consolidate the material you are learning.

QUESTIONS

1. Illustrate methods of improving memory.
2. List causes of forgetting and describe theories of forgetting.
3. Describe short-term memory and differentiate with long-term memory.
4. State process of memory (Information processing).
5. Short notes on:
    a. Childhood amnesia
    b. Memory
    c. Types of memory
    d. Short-term memory
    e. Psychological amnesia
    f. Proactive inhibition
    g. Retroactive inhibition.

11 Thinking and Reasoning

Man is differentiated from animals because of his ability to think and speak. More than two thousand years ago, Aristotle referred to man as a thinking animal. The term homosapiens used by biologists to refer to human beings, means thinking or wise men.

Thinking is a higher mental process which involves verbal symbols, internal, visual and auditory images, ideas, concepts and mathematical symbols. It takes into account past experiences, future possibilities and external realities as well. Thinking usually takes place when the individual is exposed to an unfamiliar situation in which habitual responses are inadequate for adjustment. Such a situation is known as problem situation. We conclude:

a. Thinking is a cognitive activity
b. It is goal directed
c. It is a problem solving behaviour
d. It is a process of mental exploration
e. The process of thinking involves use of symbols. A symbol represents some event or item in the world
f. Images, concepts, symbols and languages are used as instruments of thinking.

KINDS OF THINKING

1. Perceptual or Concrete Thinking

It is based on perception. Perception is the process of interpretation of sensation according to one's experience. It is also called concrete thinking as it has carried over the perception of actual or concrete objects and events. Being the simplest form of thinking, small children are mostly benefited by this type of thinking.

2. Conceptual or Abstract Thinking

It does not require the perception of actual objects or events. It is abstract thinking and makes use of concepts or abstract ideas. It is superior to perceptual thinking as it economizes efforts in understanding and helps in discovery and invention. Language plays an important part in conceptual thinking.

3. Creative Thinking

The thinking of scientists or inventors is an example of creative thinking. It is not bound by any established rule. The person himself formulates the problem and he is free to gather evidences and to invent tools for its solution. Creative thinking is aimed at creating something new.

4. Reasoning (Reflective Thinking or Logical Thinking)

Reasoning is one of the best forms of controlled thinking in which the thought process is directed consciously towards the solutions of a problem. All facts are arranged in a logical order.

Reasoning is the highest form of thinking to find out causes and predict effects. By this process, an individual tries to solve a problem by incorporating two or more aspects of his past experience. Reasoning enables to figure out the implication of certain facts or hypotheses and to derive certain generalisation.

Reasoning may be broadly classified into two types. Inductive reasoning and Deductive reasoning. Inductive logic (reasoning) arrives at a general principle based on particular instances. For example, having seen a number of crows to be black, one comes to the conclusion that all crows are black. Deductive logic (reasoning) deals with scales for drawing valid conclusions from assumptions. For example, we asssume that all men are mortal. Then we talk about a particular man say. Madhu and derive the conclusion that Madhu is mortal. Causes for making errors in reasoning are faulty fact gathering, prejudice, emotional problems, cultural barriers and fixation.

5. Problem Solving

Problem solving is an important kind of thinking. Problem solving behaviour occurs in novel or difficult situations in which a solution is not obtainable by the habitual method of applying concepts and principles derived from the past experience in a similar situation.

Problem situation occurs when there is an obstacle to reach the goal. The obstacle may be physical, social or financial which may hinder progress of the individual towards the goal.

Problem solving can be done by trial and error or mechanical means. But these methods are time consuming and hence ineffective. Problem solving can also be done through insight which is a sudden understanding which comes after studying the problem.

Scientific Method of Problem Solving

This involves seven steps (John Dewey):

1. *Recognising the problem:* It is quite possible to have a problem and not be aware of it especially in its early stages.
2. *Defining the problem:* To state exactly what this problem is, i.e. identifying the problem in definite terms.
3. *Collecting relevant information (data):* From all possible sources that have bearing on the problem. Appropriate tools are gathered, books and magazines collected.
4. *Formulation of hypothesis or possible solutions:* One tries to think of the various possibilities for the solution of the problem in the light of the information and one's own experiences. Intelligence and other cognitive abilities also help in the formulation of an appropriate hypothesis.
5. *Evaluation of the hypothesis for possible solutions:* We put into practice the course of action we have chosen as the most appropriate and varify its rightness by the results or conclusions. All tentative solutions should be closely analysed and evaluated.
6. *Verification:* The validity of the derived conclusion is tested by employing them in solution of various similar problems. If they are found suitable in solving these problems, they are accepted for the current situation also.

7. *Choosing another action if unsuccessful:* If another action is necessary you will have to return to your list of possible solutions and choose again.

If your problem is not getting good grades in the examination, it may be due to a serious health problem and you may need more extensive health care. If you have emotional problems, you may need counselling. If you have no funds for your education, you may have to apply for a scholarship. You could analyse any one of the problems listed above and find a number of reasonable solutions. The important thing is to evaluate the results, accept them as good or unsuccessful and then choose further or different action if necessary.

Another example of problem solving is that of going from one place to another place. If one recognises this problem he might use a route map, refer to sign posts, and choose one of the many possible routes depending upon what he wants. If he wants a comfortable and safe journey, he will select a national highway and so on.

Thinking and the Nurse

Nursing practice is improved by an ability to think creatively and use reliable problem solving methods. The nurse can practise good habits of thinking and systematic problem solving in the profession and all areas of her life like planning her career, problems in family life, difficulties in professional and personal relationships.

Daily problem solving is a major challenge for the nurse. It is important to have accurate data upon which to base reasoning or problem solving. Much of the data used by you will be gathered through your own observation and perception. Other data may be supplied through monitors, laboratory tests and from other members of the health team. Develop the following habits:

1. Collect as much factual information as possible
2. Beware of your own prejudices as well as those of your patients
3. Separate facts from opinion, important from minor details
4. Search carefully for underlying physical and emotional problems
5. Define the problem clearly

6. Look for relationships between cause and effect
7. Do not jump to any hasty conclusion
8. Listen to all solutions suggested by others
9. Think about all solutions suggested by others
10. Choose one solution and test to see if you have chosen the correct solution
11. Keep an open mind by constant questioning of self and others.

QUESTIONS

1. How do you define thinking?
2. Describe the steps in problem solving. Give an example of an actual nursing situation in which this process operates in full.
3. Write short notes on:
   a. Conceptual thinking
   b. Logical
   c. Creative thinking.

12 Observation: Attention, Sensation and Perception

SENSATION

Sensations are the result of physical stimuli operating on our nervous system. The process of sensing, attending and interpreting is called perception.

Various physical energies in the environment act on the sense organs. The receptors in them are stimulated from which nerve impulses are transmitted to the brain. Perception of objects and events is produced when these nerve impulses are processed.

There are eight basic sensations involving eight different sense organs and resulting in eight different types of sensory experiences (Table 12.1).

Table 12.1: Sense organs and sensory experiences

Name of the sensation	Sense organs	Sensory experience
Vision	The human eye	Light, colour, shape, form
Audition	The ear—the basillary membrane	Different sounds
Taste	The tongue—the taste buds	Sweet, sour, bitter, spicy
Olfaction	The nose—receptors in the nasal passage	Sweet, fragrant, pungent
Cutaneous	The skin	Heat, cold, pain and pressure
Kinesthetic	The muscles-receptors in the muscles	Sense of pull, push and strain
Organic	Receptors and muscles of the internal organs	Bodily sensations like hunger, thirst, nausea
Static or posture sense	Ear, semicircular canal	Sense of equilibrium, dizziness, reclining

Sensory Disorders and Defects

When the receptors are not functioning properly, we have sensory disorders or defects. The result is our false or incomplete impressions of our environment, e.g. myopia (near sightedness), hyperopia (farsightedness), astigmatism, squint and farsightedness of old age are due to deficiencies of the cornea and the lens. Colour blindness is due to retinal deficiencies.

Sensory Process and the Ward Nurse

1. A patient reacts to colours. There are some colours which are soothing. The patient who needs rest should use subdued light. For stimulation and encouragement, bright light can be used in the ward.
2. A sick person cannot tolerate loud noise and becomes irritable. The nurse should do her best in reducing the noise level in the ward.
3. Wards in a hospital often have disagreeable smells and odours. The nurse should see that the doors and windows are kept open to reduce the bad smell in the wards.
4. To help the patient relish their food, it should be warm, fresh, clean and tasty.
5. Nurses must have highly developed kinesthetic sense and should move slowly but deliberately and gracefully in the ward. Jerky movements of the nurse in the ward will result in discomfort to the patients.

ATTENTION

The first stage of perception is attention. Attention is the focusing of consciousness on a particular object or idea at a particular time, to the exclusion of other objects or ideas (Tables 12.2 and 12.3).

Types or Varieties of Attention

Our attention can be involuntary, voluntary or habitual.

1. *Involuntary attention* does not require any conscious effort to attend to an object. We give involuntary attention to loud sounds, bright lights and strong penetrating odours.
2. *In voluntary attention,* we have to make a deliberate effort, e.g. uninteresting lectures, difficult assignments.

Table 12.2: Objective conditions or external factors which increase attention (present in environment)

1. Nature of the stimulus	More attractive stimulus catches maximum attention. Pictures catch more attention than words. Coloured pictures attract more attention than black and white.
2. Location of stimulus	A stimulus in front of the eye attracts our attention more than other. In newspapers, a picture in the centre attracts more than one in a corner of the page.
3. Intensity	Loud sounds, bright colours, intense odours.
4. Change in the intensity of the stimulus	Ticking of a clock in our room may not attract our attention but when it stops, our attention is attracted. Early morning music may not awaken us if it is of constant soft volume. But we will awake if it suddenly becomes very loud or stops. Experienced speaker changes the volume of his voice while addressing an assembly.
5. Movement	A fast moving electric sign attracts our attention. Moving toys have greater appeal to children.
6. Size	Bigger size attracts more attention, but a small advertisement on a very wide background also attracts attention. Thus attention of an object does not depend on size alone, but also on the background. We notice unusually tall people or midgets.
7. Contrast	Any object different from its surroundings will stand out and attract our attention, e.g. a single man among many women, a spot on a clean white dress, a smudge on a clean wall.
8. Novelty	A new and unusual hospital equipment, a new fashion in dress.
9. Repetition	A repeated cry, repeated ringing of a call bell; certain important facts repeated by the teacher for the attention of the students; commodities are repeatedly advertised in the television; many posters of a movie are stuck on the walls for effective advertisement.

Table 12.3: Internal factors or subjective conditions of attention (present in the individuals)

Condition	Examples
Interest	When we are motivated to a goal we focus all our attention towards that goal. A sportsman eagerly looks for the sports column of the newspapers; a nurse may see news regarding employment, hospitals and new medical equipment.
Motives	When a child is hungry, he cries and looks for the feeding bottle ignoring even his favourite toys.
Experience	We attend to objects with which we are familiar what we attend to depend on selection, organisation and certain stimuli and not to all. A child when seeing an apple for the first time, does not perceive it as something to be eaten. Different people perceive the same object differently as per their experience.
Mental set or expectancy	An individual's mental set represents his feelings, attitudes, interests, habits, needs and expectation, e.g. while expecting a friend, we perceive any knocking sound as that of the friend's footsteps. In a psychological experimental, hungry students reported edible items when shown ambiguous pictures in dim light. Students who had their meals, perceived the same as play items like the bat and ball.
Emotional stage	Emotional states distort the perceptual field. Under stressful conditions we fail to perceive our surroundings fully.

3. In *habitual attention,* there is no conscious effort or sensation so striking to attract our involuntary attention. We attend to them because of our attitudes, habits or interests, e.g. the attention that a nurse gives to her patients or books on nursing arts.

Span of attention, the maximum amount of material that can be attended to in one period of attention is called "span of attention". If you are able to note five digits or five letters in a single act of attention, your span of attention is five. The number plates of motor vehicles have four digits for traffic police to notice when their span of attention is only four.

Distraction of attention refers to shifting of attention from one stimulus to another.

Examples:

- *External distraction:* Noise pollution
- *Internal distraction:* Pain, headache

Division of attention refers to the process of dividing our attention equally and simultaneously between two or more objects. For example, listening to a lecture and writing notes.

Attention may become divided and distracted. While reading a book, a student may hear his favourite song. In one case, he may stop reading and listen to the music. In the second case, he may give up the music and continue reading the book. In the third case there could be total confusion. In still another case, the student may read the book and at the same time listen to the music. Division of attention leads to the deterioration of quality and quantity of all the tasks attended simultaneously.

PERCEPTION (SENSATION PLUS INTERPRETATION)

Observation involves two mental activities—attention and perception. Perception is the interpretation of sensory stimuli which reach from the sense organs to brain. Interpretation gives meaning to sensation and we become aware of the objects.

Perception is the process by which we discriminate among stimuli and interpret their meanings and appreciate their significance, e.g. when we hear a sound, we are able to identify it as being produced by an aeroplane or an automobile. Perception gives meaning to sensation.

Human beings have perceptions corresponding to each sense organ-visual perception, auditory perception, etc.

Factors Influencing Perception

1. Functioning of the sense organs
2. Functioning of the brain
3. Previous experience
4. Frequency of exposure
5. Psychological state of the individual
6. Interest
7. Motivation
8. Behaviour of the organism.

Errors or Abnormalities in Perception

1. Illusion is wrong or false perception because of wrong interpretation of stimuli, e.g.
   a. A rope in the dark is perceived as a snake.
   b. A moving dry leaf in the dark is perceived as a moving insect.
   c. Illusion of motion picture on the screen (cinema).
   d. Judging the taste of lemon juice as that of orange juice is a gustatory illusion (Fig. 12.1).
2. Hallucination is an extreme form of inaccurate perception in which one sees something or hears some voice while nothing like that exists in the environment, e.g. perceiving a snake even in the absence of a rope, or seeing a ghost in the dark. Hallucination is felt only by those who are mentally sick or emotionally maladjusted.

   Like illusion, hallucination sometimes depends on the mental state like fear, anxiety and culture. The differences are:
   a. In illusion, there is an external stimulus which may not be present in hallucination.
   b. While illusion often happens to ordinary people, hallucination is experienced by the mentally affected, tired or intoxicated people.
3. *Imperception:* Inability to recognise due to damage to sense agains.

Abnormalities in Sensory Perception

a. *Anaesthesia* is a condition in which a person cannot respond to any sensory stimuli. It is caused by defective sense organs, drugs or emotional stress. Some organs may be abnormal due to injury or illness. Drugs are used in the operating rooms to anaesthetise a patient. We sometimes do not notice a pen or a bunch of keys lying before us and make a frantic search for it. We are either emotionally distrubed or preoccupied with some other thoughts.
b. *Hyperthesia* means excessive response to stimuli. Patients in the ward often show this behaviour. They react violently to noises

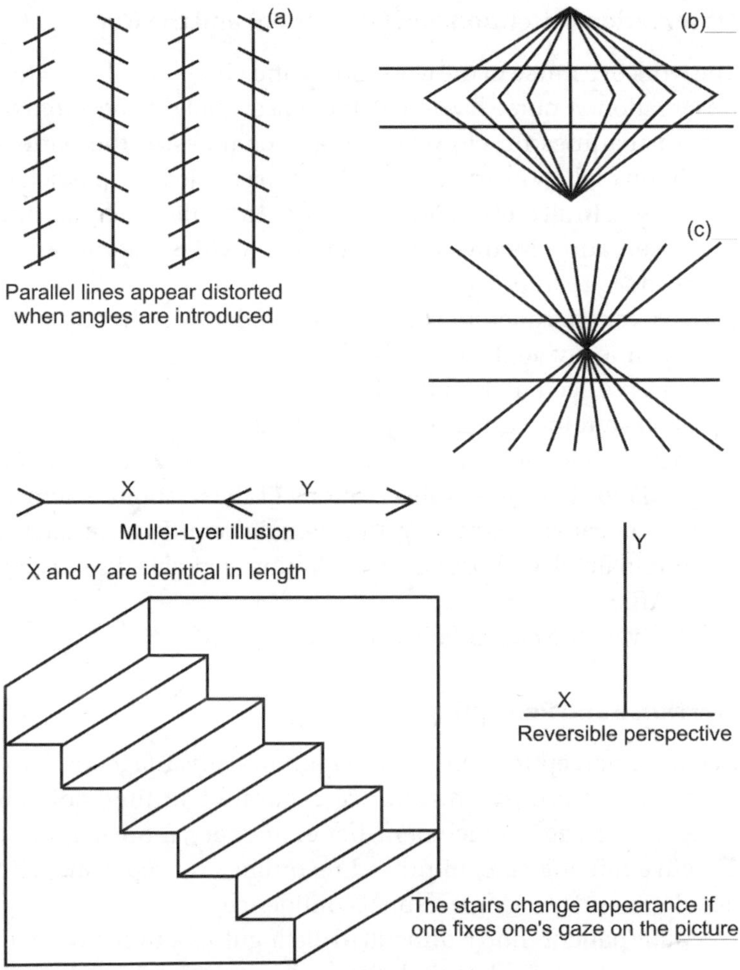

Fig. 12.1: Some examples of illusions

or bright lights. When we are fatigued, we become hyperactive to lights, to sounds or to the weight of clothing and to others.

c. *Paraesthesia* is grossly false sensation. A person of poor health or poor physiological balance may have sensations of offensive smells or bitter taste in the mouth when there is no reason for them.

Observation (Attention and Perception) and the Nurse

The work of a nurse in the classrooms and clinics involve accurate observation. A nurse has to feel the pulse, read the thermometer, record readings on charts, note any changes in the patient's conditions, follow instructions and administer doses of medicine to the patient. In all these activities, she has to be absolutely accurate.

Observation involves two mental activities—attention and perception. To improve observation:

a. Give your full attention to each task. Undertake only one activity at a time. Avoid distractions.
b. Observe accurately and quickly but not hastily.
c. Keep your interest and motivation active.
d. Avoid personal bias or prejudice. It is possible to make only partial or inaccurate observations of those about whom you have negative feelings, e.g. the mentally retarded, the aged, the terminally-ill or those with socially unacceptable diseases such as AIDS.
e. Cultivate the habit of observing accurately.

The Nurse and Perception

Accurate perception and observation are advantageous for the nurse. Some positive results are accurate learning, adjusting more quickly, good judgement, better memory, more helpful and effective nursing care, improved recording and reporting, fewer accidents and growing personal confidence.

Many patients find it difficult to distinguish between what they see and hear in the hospital. Particular attention must be given to a patient with any defect in vision or hearing, patients whose eyes are bandaged, those who are only partially aware of their environment because of sedation or those whose position in bed makes it difficult to observe what is going on. Demonstrating and allowing the patient to touch, confirming the patient's perception when he is right and correcting him when he is mistaken are essential to good nursing.

QUESTIONS

1. Distinguish observation from perception. Indicate the characteristics of perception.
2. What is attention? Discuss the internal and external determinants of attention.
3. Distinguish between illusion and hallucination?
4. What is perception? What are the organising factors in perception? Mention the perceptual disturbances. Give examples.
5. Explain the nature and characteristics of attention. Mention its types. What are the determinants of attention? Give examples.
6. Define attention. What are the determinant factors of attention? Briefly describe the types of attention.
7. Why is it important for a nurse to cultivate the habit of correct observation? What should be done to improve the accuracy of observation?
8. Sensation is the initial response of an organism to a stimulus. Perception comes a split second later and involves an interpretation or evaluation of the stimulus. Distinguish between sensation and perception, giving examples from your everyday life.
9. Describe the factors that affect the formation of our perception. What is meant by the statement "every perception is an apperception"?
10. Explain the following with examples:
    a. Anaesthesia
    b. Hyperthesia
    c. Paraesthesia
    d. Hallucination
    e. Illusion

13 Intelligence and Its Measurement

DEFINITIONS

- Intelligence is the ability to give response that are true—Thorndike
- Intelligence is the ability to carry on abstract thinking—Terman
- Intelligence is a biological adaptation consisting of the processes of assimilation and accommodation—Piaget
- Intelligence is a goal-directed behaviour—Binet
- Intelligence is creativity—Guilford

Intelligence is an individual's personality characteristic. David Wechsler suggests that intelligence of a person is his ability to adjust to the world. Wechsler has defined intelligence as the aggregate or global capacity of the individual to think rationally, to act purposefully, and to deal effectively with the environment (1958). It includes the power of adaptation of an individual to his milieu and his ability to learn and do abstract thinking.

TYPES OF INTELLIGENCE

Intelligence can be divided into three kinds:

- Mechanical intelligence
- Social intelligence
- Abstract (or general) intelligence.

Mechanical Intelligence

It is the skill to manipulate tools and gadgets and in managing the working of machines. Mechanical engineers and trained industrial workers have an abundance of mechanical intelligene.

Social Intelligence

It means understanding of people and the ability to act wisely in human relationships. Salesmen, diplomats and politicians are to be socially intelligent.

Abstract Intelligence

It is the ability to handle words, numbers, formulae and scientific principles. A person with abstract intelligence is able to discover relations among symbols to solve problems, e.g. professionals like doctors, lawyers and literary men should have abstract intelligence.

In selecting personnel for various jobs, it is useful to know the type of intelligence of the applicant.

There are differences between intelligence and aptitude. Intelligence test is the assessment of the capacity or the potentiality that a person has, whereas the aptitude tests measure capacity that predicts what one can accomplish with training. An aptitude is a combination of characteristics indicative of an individual's capacity to acquire some specific knowledge or skill. It reveals an individual's promise of essential teachability in a given area.

Spearman's Two Factor Theory of Intelligence

According to the British psychologist, Charles Spearman (1927) intelligence consists of general ability that works in conjunction with special abilities. Fundamental to all intellectual functioning is the influence of "G" or general factor but the presence of various special "S" abilities is responsible for the relationships that exist between specifically demonstrated abilities such as musical or athletic skill. Spearman thought that every test is composed of the "G" factor which is universal plus a specific "S" factor that is found in each test alone. For example, an arithmetic test might tap both "G" and "S", a specific mathematical ability. The idea that intelligence can be largely summed up with one score (e.g. IQ) is closely related to Spearman's idea that intelligence consists of one general ability factor.

Assessment of Intelligence

Alfred Binet (1875-1911) was the first psychologist to devise an intelligence test. Binet and Theodore Simon developed their first intelligence scale in 1905. Their scale consisted of 30 items arranged in order of difficulty. Their method of calculating the mental age was based on the observation that intellectual performance of a child increased with age till 18 years.

The test developed by Binet and Simon to identify mentally retarded children in French Schools served its purpose well. Subsequently, English language versions of the test were produced, e.g. by Lewis Terman of Stanford University in 1916 known as Stanford-Binet intelligence scale. In India, Binet-Kamath intelligence scale is widely used.

The test gives increasingly difficult questions for each age group because it assumes that intellectual ability in a child increases with age. Thus, there is a different test for each age group. Some examples of what would be expected of each age are given below:

Two years old:	Name various parts of the body on a paper figure.
Three years old:	Copy a drawing of a circle.
Four years old:	Explain correctly why we have houses or books.
Five years old:	Copy a drawing of a square, define words like ball or stove.
Six years old:	Can deal with numbers.
Nine years old:	Can rhyme simple words.
Adult:	Can describe the differences in meaning of abstract words.

The score of the Stanford-Binet intelligence test will give the mental age (MA).

Intelligence Quotient (IQ)

William Stern, the German psychologist introduced the concept of IQ. IQ is obtained when the mental age (MA) is divided by the chronological age (CA), which is the actual age of the person in years and multiplied by 100 (to avoid decimals):

$$IQ = \frac{MA}{CA} \times 100$$

Imagine a 10-year-old child scores a mental age of 12. His IQ will be:

$$IQ = \frac{MA}{CA} \times 100 = \frac{12}{10} \times 100 = 120$$

If a 12-year-old child scores a mental age of 12. His IQ will be:

$$IQ = \frac{MA}{CA} \times 100 = \frac{12}{12} \times 100 = 100$$

If two children both obtain an MA of 5 years, but one child is 4 years old and the other is six:

	Child 1	Child 2
$IQ = \frac{MA}{CA} \times 100$	$IQ = \frac{5}{4} \times 100 = 125$	$IQ = \frac{5}{6} \times 100 = 83$

Thus, the bright child has an IQ of 125 while the slower child has an IQ of 83.

Any person will reach a maximum IQ at about 18 years. Depending upon favourable conditions such as higher education and challenging learning experience, the IQ may increase slightly till age thirty. After 30, the IQ does not change except that it decreases slightly with old age. There is no difference between IQ of men and women.

When children grow into adults the CA will constantly increases but MA will change very little. Thus, as per the formula:

$$IQ = \frac{MA}{CA} \times 100$$

Then, IQ will become lower and lower for a person growing older and older. Therefore, the results of IQ test for adults are compared with the test results of other adults of the same age and not with the same person's chronological age. This is called the deviation IQ.

Types of Intelligence Tests

Stanford-Binet test is an individual verbal test. They have oral items. The ability of individuals on concepts like comprehension, reasoning, vocabulary, memory, etc. are measured by their verbal abilities.

Wechsler Tests

David Wechsler developed a family of tests for people at various age levels. The tests include the Wechsler adult intelligence scale revised (WAIS-R, 1981) the Wechsler preschool and primary scale of intelligence (WPPSI, 1967) for children between 6 and 16 and the Wechsler intelligence scale for children revised (WISC-R, 1974) for children between 4 to 6½ years. These are all individual tests made up of a variety of tasks.

Wechsler scales have many advantages. The administration procedures for all the three tests are similar. Scores in the subsets of these scales enable the investigator to infer patterns of abilities from which localised brain damage can be identified. Wechsler scales have been found to have even cross cultural validation.

Wechsler's tests have been adapted for Indian population. Another Indian test, *Bhatia's battery of performance* is also widely used. This test has five sub-tests namely, Koh's block design test, pass along test, pattern drawing test, immediate memory for sound and picture construction test.

When the individual tests are given to large groups, they are called group tests of the verbal type. When tests use very little language and focus on what people do with their hands they are called performance tests. These may be administered to an individual or to a large groups.

Performance tests are useful when the person being tested cannot speak the language, is deaf or dumb or has little educational background. Group testing is widely used when it is necessary to screen, many people such as those who seek admission to college, the military or various other kinds of employment.

Uses of Intelligence Testing or Uses of 'IQ'

Intelligence testing is used to predict how well a person will learn in a programme of study. They help to classify students, so that the teacher knows the capacity of each student to learn. They help to separate slower learner from the gifted learner, so that special methods can be adopted for training these two different groups. They are used in selection for admission into different courses of study and for awarding scholarships and vocational guidance. They are used in selection of candidates for different jobs.

Although intelligence tests are useful, they must be treated as guides to decisions rather than absolute statements. They do measure certain mental abilities but do not give any clue regarding a person's morals, character, emotions, general temperament and ability to work with other people.

Individual Differences in Intelligence

Intelligence (like many other psychological traits) seems to be distributed in the population in such a way that most people make score in the middle range while only a few people make very high or very low scores. This produces a bell-shaped distribution, the normal curve (Fig. 13.1).

"Individual difference" is one of the most important characteristics of intelligence. Sir Francis Galton (1883) was the first scientist to study the individual difference in a systematic way. He found that people differed from one another in their intellectual ability. The fact behind individual differences is that the two individuals differ in their genetic make up and also in the environment in which they are brought up.

There exists wide individual differences among individuals with regards to intelligence (Table 13.1). Not even identical twins or individuals matured almost in similar environment have equal intelligence (mental energy). Intelligence testing has indicated that not only there is difference in intelligence in different individuals but intelligence varies in the same individual from time to time and situation to situation.

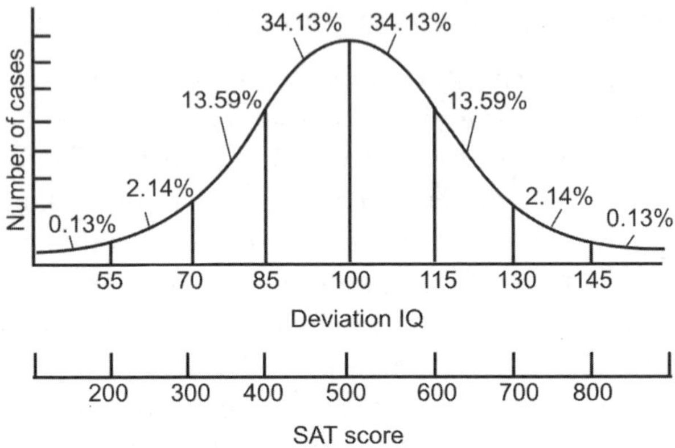

Fig. 13.1: Norms for IQ and SAT (Scholastic aptitude test) scores. Norms for large groups of measurements often approximate the normal curve (top). The numbers above the curve give the percentages of people in each in the indicated segments. For instance, 13.59 percent of the population obtain IQ scores between 115 and 130.

Table 13.1: Normal distribution of IQs for a test with a standard deviation of 15

IQ	Description	% Population
130 and above	Very superior	2.2
120–129	Superior	6.7
110–119	Bright normal	16.1
85–109	Average	59.1
70–84	Borderline	13.6
55–69	Mildly mentally retarded	2.1
40–54	Moderately mentally retarded	0.1
25–39	Severely mentally retarded	0.003
Below 25	Profoundly mentally retarded	0.0000005

Intelligence and sex difference: Various studies have been conducted to find out whether there is any difference in the intelligence levels of males and females. In most cases, no significant differences have been noticed. Therefore, differences in sex does not contribute towards differences in intelligence. If at all, women prefer particular subjects for study, it may be explained as due to their aptitude.

Intelligence and racial or cultural differences: Earlier studies in USA which indicated the whites to be a superior race to the Blacks have been questioned. Present indications are that intelligence does not depend on the race or group. The "bright" and the "dull" can be found in any race or caste or cultural group and the differences are due to the influence of environment.

Heredity and Environment

Studies of monozygotic twins (twins originated from the same ovum) reared in different environment had shown high similarities in behaviour and intelligence which emphasises the role of heredity.

Emotional deprivation due to parental rejection, traumatic experiences like death of beloved ones and separation from parents can affect the mental functioning of individuals. Lack of opportunities affects language development, problem solving skills and coping skills which in turn affects intellectual functioning. Even malnutrition has adverse effects on mental functioning. All these suggest the influence of environment on intelligence.

Children from lower social class families generally perform less well on intelligence test than from higher social class. Greater parental attention received by children of smaller families and the first borns may result in higher IQ scores.

Success of attempts through intensive stimulation and education to improve the IQ in high risk children and mentally handicapped demonstrate the importance of environment.

Similarly IQ scores have been found to increase when children are transferred from poor institutions to good foster homes.

Heredity has been compared to seed and environment to land. Just as fertile land and good quality seeds are required for good crop, both good heredity and stimulating environment are required for higher intelligence.

Both heredity and environment affect intelligence. The nature nurture controversy is regarding the relative importance of these factors. Intelligence can be raised by improving the environment in such areas as education and living conditions. In this case, the limit of how far intelligence can be raised would be set by the inherited level of intelligence. Intelligence could be lowered to any depth if malnutrition, poverty and poor living condition existed far long periods. Many suffer from mental retardation and low level of intelligence in countries where millions have starved to death and millions have suffered severe malnutrition.

Any person will reach a maximum intelligence (IQ) at about age eighteen. It is possible to have a slight increase of IQ until one is almost thirty. This increase depends upon favourable conditions such as higher education or challenging learning experience. IQ changes very little after thirty years of age except to go down slightly in the advanced age.

Causes of Mental Retardation or Subnormality (IQ below 70)

The causes of mental retardation are often unknown. About 25 percent of all cases are due to physical disorders such as:

1. Birth injuries which are often due to lack of oxygen or caused by an extremely difficult birth
2. Total damage as from use of drugs by the mother or infections of the mother before birth of the child or immediately after birth
3. Metabolic disorders
   a. Phenylketonuria
   b. Cretinism
4. Genetic abnormalities
   a. Down's syndrome
   b. Cerebral palsy.

Management of the Retarded or Mentally Subnormal (IQ below 70)

Retarded individuals take longer to learn new material and once they have learned something new, they usually forget more easily than do the normal persons. They need more sympathetic help from parents and teachers for learning skills. They often fail to learn by observation and, therefore, need more structured teaching. Help needs to be provided at an appropriate level for the child. It is useless to try and teach skills too far ahead of the child's present mental age. In the preschool period, the main task of professional teachers and speech therapists is in helping the parents to find ways to stimulate their child's development.

The Mentally Gifted Children (IQ above 140)

These are children with IQs 140 and above. In the early childhood, a gifted child is generally found to be a misfit in his class because the level of teaching in normal class room is for average child, whereas the gifted child is able to comprehend must faster. As a consequence, they lose interest in studies and indulge in behavioral irregularities. They become gross underachievers and extremely unhappy. They find themselves intellectually misfit with children of their age and physically misfit with older people who are their intellectual equal. But things improve by adulthood and they appear to be happier and better adjusted than most others of their age.

It is important to recognise a gifted child. Parents and teachers should be aware of the child who wants everything explained, solves problems easily, has an exceptional memory, talks in complete senstences at as early as two years of age, and is clever with the hands such as mechanical, musical and artistic abilities. With the right type of training, their superior potential should be channelised in constructive tasks. Some school systems provide special classes and programmes for the mentally gifted as well as mentally retarded.

Intelligence and the Nurse

Knowledge of intellectual functioning is useful to a student nurse and later on for her as a teacher. Teaching methods, content of the subject matter and student expectations will be based on the intelligence level of the class.

Assessment and understanding of intellectual functions will be helpful to the nurse in her clinical work. She would be able to diagnose a patient with mental subnormality or with superior intelligence. Her explanations or guidance to the patients and their families would be according to their IQ. In diseases like neuropsychiatric disorders, epilepsy, psychiatric disorders and in some endocrinal disorders, assessment of intelligence is of great assistance in their management.

Understanding the development of intelligence in babies and children is another challenge for the nurse. Babies and children should be closely observed for abnormalities and for very high or very low intelligence levels. When caring for older children, it is important to undertand how the child's intelligence develops with years. The mildly mentally retarded will respond and accept responsibility for themselves if they are given the right kind of encouragement, environment and an opportunity to learn.

Recognising individual levels of intelligence in your different professional colleagues and co-workers is also important in communicating with them. It will be the nurse's responsibility to know when communications or instructions can be given quickly in professional terms or when they must be given in simple terms and possibly repeated until well understood.

QUESTIONS

1. Explain the terms "heredity" and "environment". What roles do they play in the development of the individual?
2. Explain the meaning of "Intelligence". What are the various types of intelligence tests? Mention their uses.
3. Define the term mental sub-normality. What is the role of nurse in helping parents of a mentally retarded child.
4. Define the term "Individual differences". Mention the causes of individual differences. Explain the role of teachers in educating slow learners.
5. Explain the meaning of intelligence. What is the nature of distribution of intelligence? How is intelligence measured?
6. Define IQ. What is the current status of IQ and intelligence tests?

14 Personality and Its Development

"Let me have men about me that are fat; sleek-headed men and such as sleep o'nights. Yond Cassius has a lean and hungry look; He thinks too much. Such men are dangerous".

—Shakespeare's Julius Caeser

The word personality is derived from Greek word "*Persona*" the mask used by actors in Greek drama.

Personality is the total quality of an individual's behaviour as it is shown in his habits of thinking, in his attitude, interests, his manner of acting and his personal philosophy of life. It is the totality of his being. Personality is more than the sum total of an individual's traits and characteristics. It is expressed through his behaviour. The characteristic combinations of behaviour distinguish one individual from another giving each a unique personality and identify.

Personality is often confused with character and temperament. Character means a judgement of individual based upon certain qualities. A person has a good or bad character depending on whether or not he is honest and dependable. Character reflects the part of the personality related to one's value system.

Temperament is the hereditary emotional aspects of personality. We refer to a person's temperament as "irritable and fuzzy", "moody" or "sensitive".

Components of Personality

1. *Physical:* These are the physical traits or features of an individual namely, height, weight, colour, expression facial physical health. In general, a good personality means an impressive, symmetrical and healthy body.

2. *Emotional:* A person's emotions also go into the make up of his personality.
3. *Intelligence:* An intelligent person will have a forceful personality. A person with subnormal intelligence is a "dull" person.
4. *Behaviour:* Behaviour is a reflection of one's personality. It is partly dependent on our feelings and partly on the expectations of the society. Behaviour may be gentle, kind, affectionate, balanced, submissive or aggressive.

DEVELOPMENTAL THEORIES

There are a number of approaches for studying the human development. There are several theories or set of principles of personality development which have been developed to explain personality differences. Some focus upon the internal growth of personality, others are based on the effect of one's external environment and still others emphasise personal experience and growth of self-image.

Psychoanalytical Theory

Sigmund Freud (1856–1936) developed the best known theory of personality focussed upon internal growth or psychodynamics.

I. Structure of Personality

Freud thought of personality as being based upon a structure of three parts: The Id, the ego and the superego (Fig. 14.1).

The id is composed of biological instincts including the drives of sex and aggression. It is self-centred, impulsive but unconscious. All the drives of a person towards pleasure and self-satisfaction are coming from the Id. This uninhibited demand for self-satisfaction is called the pleasure principle. Id does not bother about the environment, the needs of others or reality but demands complete self-satisfaction. An infant is all id as it demands immediate satisfaction of its basic needs like hunger, thirst, relief from discomfort or pain without concern for how it will be done immediately.

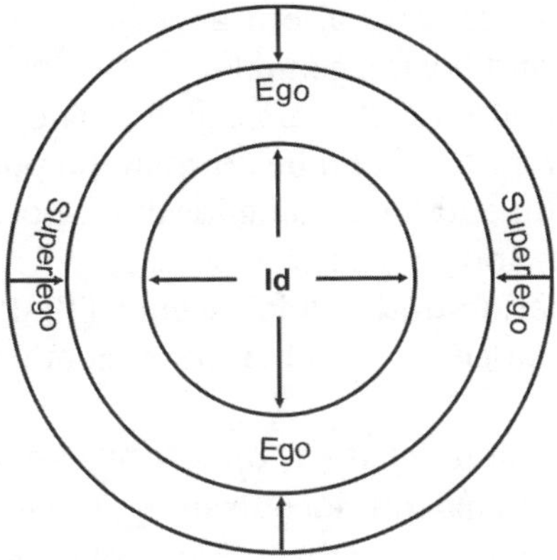

Fig. 14.1: Id, ego, superego

The ego called self, gets energy from the id but serves as a control for the Id through its contact with reality. Ego directs the behaviour of personality through the reality principle. Many demands of id are not realistic and hence will be controlled by the ego.

The superego is made up of the conscience and the ego ideal. It is developed through the cultural environment and learning from social contacts such as parents, family members and authority figures. It judges the thoughts and actions of the ego. When a person behaves against the standards of his superego (= conscience) he will feel guilty.

Freud believed that the id, ego and superego are in constant conflict with one another, the ego controlling the demands of the id and the superego checking the behaviour of the ego.

II. Psychosexual Stages

According to Freud, all human beings pass through a series of five psychosexual stages:

- *The oral stage* from birth to one year-pleasure is obtained through stimulation of the mouth as in nursing or thumb sucking.
- The anal stage occurring during the second year of life when toilet training is attempted—gratification is obtained through holding or expelling faeces.

- The phallic stage from about age three to six-pleasure is obtained by fondling the genitals.
- A latency period 6 to 12 years called latency because sexual interests are repressed and lie dormant till puberty. Period of gang formation and fierce gang loyalties. Boys cling together and shun girls and girls despise boys.
- The genital period during adolescence (12–19 years). Young people begin experiencing romantic infatuation and emotional unheavals.

Problems encountered at any one stage, either of deprivation or overindulgence, may produce fixation at that stage. A person fixated at the oral stage when the infant is totally dependent upon others for satisfaction of needs may, as an adult, be excessively dependent and overly fond of such oral pleasures as eating, drinking or smoking. A person fixated at the anal stage may be abnormally concerned with cleanliness and orderliness Obsessive Compulsive Disorders (OCD).

For Freud, the first six years of childhood are most critical for personality development. What happens to the individual in later life is fashioned during the child's first six years.

III.Personality Dynamics

Topographical Description of Psyche or Mind or Levels of Consciousness

Mind is a function of the body; it does not exist apart from the body. It is the sum total of the various mental processes or activities. Mental processes can be conscious, unconscious or preconscious.

The conscious: As per Freud, the conscious part of the mind consists of those mental activities of which we are aware, such as thoughts, feelings and sensations. It functions only when the individuals is awake. It directs the individuals as he behaves in a rational way.

The unconscious: The unconscious is by far the largest part of the mind. It includes our repressed desires, our fears and phobias (for which we do not know the reasons) and many others. Material stored in the unconscious has a powerful influence on our thoughts or feelings (unconscious motivation).

The preconscious or subconscious: It is the part of the mind, in which ideas and reactions are stored and partially forgotten. The preconscious also prevents certain unacceptable, disturbing unconscious memories from reaching the conscious mind. Materials from the subconscious can be brought to the conscious, if the individual concentrates on recall.

Mind and body interact on each other. Our nervous system and glands are responsible for our ways of thinking, feeling and wishing. Our feelings or our emotions can cause bodily illnesses.

Psychosocial Theory

This theory was developed by Eric Erickson (1902–1994). He challenged Freud's theory that personality is primarily established during the first six years and said that the personality continues to develop over the entire life. Individuals develop a healthy personality by mastering inner and outer dangers with positive solutions to life's problems (Table 14.1).

Cognitive Theory

The Swiss psychologist Jean Piaget (1896–1980) has proposed four main stages of intellectual or cognitive development (Table 14.2).

The quality of one's problem solving abilities and one's ability to be creative in meeting life's challenges depend upon one's ability to think. However, while cognitive theory focuses narrowly on the development of intellect and reasoning, other theories such as Erickson's involve a much broader range of human experiences.

Humanistic Theory

When personality development focusses upon the development of self, it is called humanism. Humanists like Carl Rogers and Abraham Maslow reject the internal conflicts of Freud's view and

Table 14.1: Erickson's eight life stages

Age	Stage	Central issue	Significant relations
0–18 months (infancy)	Trust vs Mistrust	Testing of the trust worthiness of the infant's significant others	Mother
18 months–3 years (early childhood)	Autonomy vs shame and doubt	Testing of the individual capabilities in relation to significant others	Parents
3–5 years (middle childhood)	Initiative vs guilt	Testing out abilities to compete in the outside world	Basic family
5–12 years (late childhood)	Industry vs inferiority	Gaining mastery of cultural tools	School
13–19 years (adolescence)	Identity vs role diffusion	Developing a sense of personal identity	Peer groups
20–30 years (early adulthood)	Intimacy vs isolation	Merging of identity with another to achieve intimacy	Friends
30–65 years (mature adult-hood or middle age)	Generativity vs stagnation	Investing creative energies in promoting social welfare	Household
65–Death (old age)	Ego integrity vs despair	Acceptance of the life one has lived as worthwhile	Mankind

Table 14.2: Piaget's four stages of congnitive development

Approximate age	Stage	Occurrences
1. Birth to 18 months	Sensory motor	Object permansence
2. 18 months to 5–6 years	Preoperational	Governed by immediate and partial percept. Egocentric thought. Cannot attend to all relevant dimensions of a problem.
3. 7 to 12–13 years	Concretely operational	Conservation of quantity and numbers. Conservation of weight and volume. Conservation of length, distance and area. No more self-centered
4. 14 years and above	Formally operational	Operations are more numerous and on a more general basis

the mechanistic nature of behaviourism. They believe that each person is creative and responsible, free to choose and each strives for fulfilment or self-actualisation.

CLASSIFICATION OF PERSONALITY

1. By types
2. By traits or factors.

Types of Personality

Types based on temperament:
Hippocrates (about 400 BC), the father of medicine, classified people into four types depending on which body fluid is predominent:

- Sanguine—cheerful (blood)
- Phlegmatic—calm (mucus)
- Choleric—irritable (Yellow bile)
- Melancholic—depressed (Black bile)

William Sheldon divided people into three types according to body build:

- Endomorph—Soft, fat and round—sociable and relaxed.
- Mesomorph—Heavy and muscular—physically active and noisy.
- Ectomorph—Tall, thin and flat-chested—self-conscious, shy and reserved.

Classification by Psychological Types

On the basis of sociability Dr Carl G Jung classified people into two main groups namely, extroverts and introverts.

Extroverts are people who take more interest in others and like to move with people and are skilled in etiquette. They are friendly and sociable and not easily upset by difficulties. They are dominated by emotions, whereby they take decisions quickly and act on them without delay. They are realistic and face the problems of life objectively.

Introverts are those who are interested in themselves, their own feelings, emotions and reactions. They are busy in their own thoughts and are self-centred. They are reserved and like to work alone. They are very sensitive and are unable to adjust easily to social situations. They are inclined to worry and easily get embarrassed. Poets, philosophers, scientists and artists belong to this group.

There are very few people who are pure extroverts or introverts. Majority of the people are ambiverts having the qualities of extroverts and introverts in different proportions.

Personality traits: The most common way to describe people, say a nurse, is to list a number of qualities she should possess, e.g. patience, honesty, perseverance, thoroughness and initiative. These qualities are called personality traits. Groups of personality traits are known as personality factors or dimensions of personality.

Factors of Personality

1. The physiological factors include the physique of the individual—his size, strength, looks and constitution.
2. The environmental or social factor.
3. Mental or psychological factors including motives, interests, attitudes, will and character, intellectual capacities as intelligence, reasoning, attention, perception and imagination. These traits and factors are assessed by psychological tests.

Assessment of Personality

The following methods are used for evaluation and assessment of personality traits:
1. Observational methods (The interview)
2. Personality inventories (Based on trait theories)
3. Projective techniques (Based on psychoanalytical theory).

Interviews: Interview is the most popular method of observation. Appearance, bearing and speech can be noticed. Questions can be asked about attitudes and interests. Interviews are used to evaluate a person's personality for the purpose of employment and for education as well as for identifying personality traits. An interview may be informal or unstructured. It can be formal or structured, where specific topics are selected by the interviewer before and the flow of conversation is controlled.

Body language of the client can be observed during an interview. The body language may be posture, movement of the hands, facial expressions or voice. However, interviews take place under stress and great skill is needed to put the interviewee at ease.

Questionnaires: This is the most common written method of assessing personality. A personality interview is a questionnaire in which the person reports his or her feeling in certain situations. They are very easily checked and scored. More often the answers are scored by machines which eliminate the prejudice of the tester, making the test more objective (Table 14.3).

Minesota Multiple Personality Inventory (MMPI): One of the most commonly used personality tests is the MMPI. This test asks for answers of "True", "False" or "Cannot" to 566 statements about different personality traits such as attitudes, emotional reactions, physical and psychological symptoms and past experiences. The answers are quantitatively measured and personality assessment is done based on the norm scores.

Personality questionnaires are used in psychology for counselling and research. They are used for selection for employment or promotion.

Projective tests: Projective tests focus upon what is inside a person rather than what can be seen in a person's behaviour. These tests try to find out more about a person's feelings, unconscious desires and inner thoughts.

Table 14.3: Examples of questions used in questionnaires

Questions	Answers	
a. Would you rate yourself as a quiet person?	Yes	No
b. Do you prefer to work alone rather than with others?	Yes	No
c. Do you frequently feel sad?	Yes	No

These tests make use of people's tendencies to make up stories about things they see. When shown an inkblot, for example, people see butterflies, dancing girls, pictures of skeletons, or many other images. When a vague picture is shown depicting two people, a story can be made about their relationship to each other, their difficulties and troubles. The stories people make up about pictures reveal something about their own personality. They project unto the picture, feelings and thoughts of their own.

The Rorschach inkblot test was the first projective test and is still widely used. It was developed by the Swiss psychologist Hermann Rorschach in 1920. Another projective test is the Thematic apperception test (TAT) developed by Henry Murray of Havard University in 1938. The Rorschach test uses ten different kinds of inkblots which must be described by the person taking the test. The TAT uses twenty sketches about which the person is asked to make up a story.

Projective tests are often used in clinical practice. They are helpful in showing a person's inner areas of conflict, anxieties or any problems in relationships because the person is free to describe anything.

In nursing, suitable pictures can be devised to test attitudes to patients, work or hospital.

Personality and the Nurse

An understanding of personality will help the nurse to predict her behaviour as well as the behaviour of others. Major decisions of life depend upon this knowledge, e.g. selection of a career, spouse, colleagues. Her relationships with friends and relatives depend upon her expectations of their behaviour from an understanding of their personalities.

A successful nurse will have a strong and pleasing personality. Besides possessing such professional qualities as integrity, dignity, mental abilities, poise, self-confidence and dependability, she must have personal qualities like sympathy, understanding friendliness and adaptability. Patients appreciate a nurse who brings physical comfort to them with her skills and who understands their emotional difficulties, caused by illness. The nurse must also have good health, fresh and neat appearance, will power, high standards of moral values, sense of humour, teaching and managerial capabilities, self-control and friendly interpersonal relationships.

QUESTIONS

1. Define personality. Describe the various types of personality.
2. Write brief notes on:
   a. Assessment of personality
   b. Structure of personality
   c. Levels of consciousness
   d. Clinical interviews.
3. What do psychologists mean by the term "personality"? In your opinion what is the role of personality in sickness and recovery?
4. Enumerate the methods of assessment of personality. Explain any two of them.
5. Examine personality. Mention its classifications. Bring out the importance of any one classification.
6. Describe the psychological classification of personality by Carl G Jung.

15 Developing Personality: Different Age Groups

CHARACTERISTICS OF VARIOUS AGE GROUPS

Childhood: Phallic Stage or the Period of Family Triangle-initiative vs Guilt (3 to 6 Years)

The pleasurable sensations have now shifted from the mouth and excretory organs to the genitals. The child will now unconsciously wish to identify with parent of the same sex and unconsciously wish to replace that parent in the family.

During this period, the little boy who always had a great deal of attention and love from his mother, begins to feel very possessive towards the mother. He wants her for himself and resents the close tie that he feels exists between his father and mother. He develops competitive feelings towards his father and tries to be rival with him for his mother's love. The father, however, is such a large and formidable opponent that the little boy develops resentment and fear of him. This is Oedipus complex.

Eventually, the little boy concludes that being like his father is more effective way of obtaining his mother's love and attention. Thus, he begins to take on the masculine behaviour of his father. This is identification. Similarly, the little girl identifies herself with the mother. Thus, the basic future relationships with men and women is initiated during this period. If for any reason, parents are people with whom the child cannot identify, future adjustment may be seriously affected. The child needs warmth, comfort, acceptance, nourishment as well as love and protection from both the parents. Both parents should have interest in their children, pride in their achievement, sympathy in their problems. Discipline is through patience, affection, understanding and reasoning. Child is respected as a person and is given freedom to develop. His early mistakes are recognised as part of "growing up." Children have respect for parents—respect-based on love and not on fear.

Puberty and Adolescence: Identity vs Role Confusion (12 to 18 Years)

The transition period from childhood to adulthood is known as adolescence. Through physical, social and mental changes, the child must develop into an adult. Caught between dependency of childhood and independence of adulthood, the teenager is strongly ambivalent in his desires and emotions. This is a trying period for him as well as his parents.

Physical changes: Towards the end of later childhood, sexual changes or puberty begins. Secondary sexual characteristics develop—enlarged hips and breasts develop in girls and muscular development and voice changes in boys. Both sexes begin to grow pubic hair. Puberty is completed when primary sexual functioning occurs.

Social changes: Life is in a state of disequilibrium. Every aspect of life is likely to be characterized by stress, storm and turmoil as the young individual attempts to become completely free from his family. Because of this conflict over dependency-independency needs, the adolescent may be hostile towards adults, particularly parents and teachers and rebellious towards authority. He craves for love, recognition and encouragement.

Development task at the adolescent stage is to develop a sense of identity regarding occupational, familial and social roles as opposed to the development of role confusion. This requires a stable, loving home-life and wise, mature parents who understand the needs of their children and treat them as individuals. The adolescent, during the stage of identity formation is likely to suffer from a confusion of roles or identity crisis. This state causes one to feel isolated, empty, anxious and indecisive. Helping adolescents feel good about themselves will promote a good nurse-patient relationship.

Mature Adulthood or Middle Age: Generativity vs Stagnation (30 to 65 Years)

People find themselves in a crisis leading to increased rate of divorces and major shift in career plans, e.g. a woman who has been satisfied as a housewife for the past 15 or 20 years may feel that she had been left out of the mainstream of life and so may take up a job. A father and husband may think that he has made a mistake not only in the choice of the job but also in the marriage partner, habits and place of residence. The mid-forties usher in the "deadline decade" (35–45), the cross-roads of life.

At the mid-forties, the equilibrium is regained. Children take up a job away from home or are married. Parents have to redefine their roles in relationship to one another, to their family and to the large world outside the family. They become involved in work outside the family. For example, a nurse who has been both a mother and nurse, may become increasingly involved in giving leadership in professional nursing. She may become involved in a group that is deciding whether nurses should strike, her attention moving from merely doing her job to broader issues of social justice.

Changes that occur during adulthood have given rise to various expressions such as "middle age", "mid-career crisis", "middle age slump"–referring to recognition of losing youth and coming of old age. Individuals become aware of ageing process and realize that time is moving on.

The conflict within this period is between generativity and stagnation. We begin to look at what we have generated-products and ideas, the legacy we leave to future generations. When generativity is weak and not given expression, the personality regresses or stagnates.

Individuals unable to make the transitions of this period, will be frightened of growing old, rather than enjoying a new type of fulfilment as they grow old. Energies are invested in holding back the tide of time, e.g. the middle-aged woman dressing like a young girl.

Old Age or Senescent: Ego Integrity vs Despair (65 Years to Death)

This period is characterized by integrity. According to Erikson, integrity sums up our ability to live the later portion of life with dignity and a sense of order and meaning to life. It involves a continued joy in living, a sense of accomplishement, of things well done. Integrity is the acceptance of one's life cycle. Despair expresses the feeling that what has been done is not of much value and that not much time is left to do anything. While looking back, if he feels that his life was successful, then he has integrity; otherwise despair.

It is necessary to adjust to the reduced income and deteriorating health. Frequently friends or husband/wife die leading to loneliness.

Nurse and the Adult Patients

Listening to the worries and concerns about family and work responsibility in both the young and middle adulthood is most helpful. Physical signs of stress should be noted. The adult should be assisted to become independent until able to assume responsibility for his or her own health.

Older adults will be hospitalized more than any other group. The elderly need warmth and personal touch of others and should be helped to prevent social isolation. They have a special need to be respected and valued as a person. They should be helped to take food, dressed and protected from cold by covering with blankets. The nurse should help the elderly hear and see more easily. Also they should be physically protected especially if disoriented.

Generally, old people become impatient and show irritability and willfulness. The nurse should realise that these are due to the normal deteriorating process. It is necessary to keep old people interested in life and make them feel important and useful.

QUESTIONS

1. Discuss the most important principles of nursing care of
   a. Children,
   b. Adolescents,
   c. The adults, and
   d. The old. Account for the differences in the care.

16 Will and Character

WILL

Will is the mental capacity of an individual to choose or decide or to do one thing rather than the other. It is the deliberate action in the line of maximum resistance. Will is required when a choice has to be made between two modes of action, between two motives, between two or more conflicting behaviour.

Will has three steps namely, deliberation, vacillation and decision. While engaged in deliberation, the individual who has to decide examines the merits and demerits of the different alternatives available to him. Sometimes the alternatives may be simple and making the choice relatively easy. But on many occasions the decision-making is difficult and completed on the alternation of equal attraction and strong repulsion. There is suspense, hesitation and vacillation and the process is personally painful. After a lot of postponement, a decision in taken at the long last, resolving the conflict between the motives.

Decision is arrived at as a result of rational thinking or by some accidental circumstance or by impulse. The decision is not due to will: In a willed decision, the whole self-consisting of ideals, sentiments and attitudes or character is in action. The whole mind in at work, not any particular motive. That is why will is often referred to as character in action.

CHARACTER

Character is one of the acquired factors of human personality, an aspect of our behaviour like habits, skills and attitudes. It is a long-lasting mental structure influencing our conduct and social behaviour. It is a mental organisation behind all our activities.

We are not born with character. It is an acquired quality. We are born with our physiological and other motives, drives and temperament. Gradually, we develop skills, habits and attitudes. All these acquired tendencies put together, give rise to a consistency of behaviour or integrated conduct which is called character. Character is the result of growth.

Character means a judgement of the individual based on certain qualities. A person has a good or bad character depending on whether or not he is honest and dependable. Character reflects the part of the personality related to one's value system.

Our character will be normally strong or good if moral ideals or sentiments have been incorporated in it. In other words, if we have formed or acquired some moral attitudes. These acquired attitudes enable us to perform acts which are normally and socially approved as desirable.

Character and will are related. If we have a strong character, we have abundant will power and no conflicts. There is no vacillation and decision are taken without delay.

Character is the mental and moral equipment acquired form education and environment. It is revealed in the conduct of the individual and his relations with others. A nurse needs to develop a character, which is both psychologically strong and morally good. Besides such professional qualities as integrity, dignity, mental abilities, poise, self-confidence and dependability, a successful nurse must acquire many moral qualities like sincerity, honesty, truthfulness and service. We include in our concept of character, both its psychological strength and moral goodness.

QUESTIONS

1. (a) Give the meaning of Will.
   (b) Mention the factors and conditions to willing.
   (c) List down six conditions which facilitate a decision.

PART—II

SOCIOLOGY

17. Definition, Scope and Methods: Importance of Sociology in Nursing
18. Culture and Community Health
19. The Individual: Growth and Development
20. Fundamental Rights and Fundamental Duties
21. The Family
22. Family Life Education
23. Social Groups
24. Social Changes and Social Control
25. Social Stratification: Rural and Urban Society
26. Social Problems
27. Social Agencies and Remedial Measures
28. Community and Culture
29. Social Security
30. Population Explosion
31. Health Economics
32. Budgeting for a Family

17 Definition, Scope and Methods: Importance of Sociology in Nursing

Auguste Compte (1798–1857), the French philosopher is traditionally considered the "father of sociology". In 1839, Compte coined the word sociology in his famous work "Positive Philosophy". The term sociology is derived from the Latin word SOCIUS, meaning companion or associate and the Greek word LOGOs meaning study or science. Thus, sociology is the science of society. Society is the largest permanent group of people with a common interest, land and way of life. Sociology is a science of society and social problems. The teaching of sociology as a separate discipline started in USA in 1876, in France in 1889, in Britain in 1907 and in India in 1919 (Bombay University).

Some prominent sociologists of India like GS Ghurye, RK Mukherjee, DP Mukherjee, Humayun Kabir, DN Mazumdar, MN Srinivas, MS Gore, PN Prabhu and AR Desai have further enriched the subject with their social investigations and writings. India, with its diverse cultural peculiarities provides wonderful opportunities for sociological research and studies.

Definition of Sociology

"Science of social phenomena, subject to natural and invariable laws, the discovery of which is the object of investigation" —Auguste Compte

"Science which attempts to the interpretative understanding of social action in order thereby to arrive at casual explanation of its cause and effects" — Max Weber

"Science of social institutions"—Emile Durkhelm

"Science of social relationships"—AW Small

"Study of social life"—Ogburn and Nimkoff

"General science of society"—Kingsby

"Sociology is the study of collective behaviour"—Park and Burgess

"Sociology is the study of human interactions and inter-relations, their conditions and consequences"—Morris Ginseburg.

We can sum up:

Sociology is the science of society.

Sociology is the study of social life.

Sociology is the study of social systems.

Sociology is the study of social relationships.

Sociology is the study of behavioural groups.

The above definitions highlight various aspects of sociology. The divergent views about the definition of sociology only reveal their different approaches to its study. However, the common idea underlying all these definitions is that sociology is concerned with man, his social relations and his society. Sociology includes various aspects of society like social interactions, relationships, institutions, groups, social processes, norms and values. Different social sciences study only a part of social behaviour. For example, political science discusses political behaviour; economics discusses economic behaviour. Thus, sociology is a general social science whereas other social sciences are special sciences of society.

Nature and Characteristics of Sociology

Robert Bierstedt in his book, "Social Order" has mentioned the following characteristics of sociology:

1. Sociology is an independent science. It is not studied as a part of any other subject like philosophy or psychology. Its subject matter has well defined boundaries and methods of study.
2. Sociology is a social science and not a physical science.

Knowledge

Physical sciences	Medical sciences	Social sciences	Humanities
E.g. 1. Physics	E.g. 1. Nursing	E.g. 1. History	E.g. 1. Arts
2. Chemistry	2. Psychiatry	2. Economics	2. Languages
3. Geology	3. Clinical psychology	3. Sociology	3. Communication
4. Geography		4. Culture	4. Speech
5. Astronomy			

Fig. 17.1: Classification of knowledge

3. Sociology is a categorical and not a mormatic discipline. It concerns itself to statements about what is, and not what should be or ought to be. It does not make any value judgements.
4. Sociology is a pure science and not an applied science. The main aim of pure sciences is the acquisition of knowledge and not its application. The immediate aim of sociology is the acquisition of knowledge about human society and not its application (Fig. 17.1).
5. Sociology is relatively an abstract science and not a concrete science. Thus, sociology is not interested in the concerete manifestation of human events. It is more concerned with the form of social events and their patterns. For example, sociology is not concerned with any particular war or revolution but with wars and revolutions in general, as social phenomena, as types of social conflicts.
6. Sociology is a general social science and not a special social science.
7. Sociology is both a rational and empirical science. The empirist collects facts and the rationalist coordinates and arranges them.

Sociology has been studied in one form or other from the time of Aristotle. In the beginning, it was a part of philosophy. Gradually, it grew into an independent subject. Recently with the increased use of scientific methods, it has developed into a positive science. Sociology, enjoys a pre-eminent position in the family of social sciences. A knowledge of sociology is considered essential in the fields of medicine, nursing, law, business, social relations, administration, social work and other areas of human endeavour.

Methods of Sociology

1. Experimental or scientific method which consists of:
   a. Formulation of hypothesis
   b. Plan of research design
   c. Collection of data
   d. Analysis of data
   e. Drawing conclusions
2. Historical method.
3. Comparison or anthropological method.
4. Questionnaire and interview method.
5. Social survey method.
6. Case history method.
7. Sociometry.

Scope or Subfields/Branches of Sociology

Sociology is a fast growing academic discipline. It has developed various subfields to study different aspects of man's social life. Each subfield employs its own approach and techniques. Some of the main branches of sociology are:

1. Rural sociology.
2. Industrial sociology.
3. Urban sociology.
4. Sociology of education.
5. Sociology of family.
6. Sociology of law.
7. Sociology of religion.
8. Sociology of occupation.
9. Cultural sociology.
10. Political sociology.

In addition, sociology has made intensive studies in many other fields like social stratification, mass media of communication, public opinion and bureaucracy. The horizon of sociology is expanding and the possibilities are endless. Gradually, it will cover man's entire social life.

Sociology and Social Psychology

The unit of study of psychology is the individual and the unit of study of sociology in the group. Social psychology is the science of the individual in society It studies the individual in group, crowd, mob, audience and other social situations. It also studies the attitudes of the individual towords cultural and social values (Table 17.1).

Table 17.1: Differences between sociology and social psychology

Sociology	Social psychology
Sociology studies society and social groups. It has no primary interest in the individual or in his personality or in his individual behaviour.	Social psychology studies the behaviour of the individual in groups, situations or in society. The focus of interest is in the individual and not the society as such.
Sociology analyses social processes.	Social psychology analyses the mental processes of man.
Sociology is interested in the social forms and structures within which the behaviour of man takes place.	Psychology and social psychology are primarily concerned with the behaviour of individual as such.
Sociology studies the groups themselves and the larger social structure within which both individual and group processes occur.	Psychology studies the individual and social psychology the individual in his social group.
Sociology studies society from the sociological point of view.	Social psychology studies the individual's behaviour from the viewpoint of the psychological factors involved

Importance of Sociology or Uses of Sociology

1. Sociology studies society in a scientific way. Scientific knowledge about human society is needed for progress in various fields of human endeavour.
2. Sociology improves our understanding of society, social groups, social institutions and their functions; and changing trends help us lead an effective and meaningful social life.

3. Sociology helps us to become broad minded by overcoming our prejudices, misconceptions, egoism, class and communal hatred.
4. Sociology helps us to understand social problems by studying their causes and solutions.
5. Social planning has been made easier by sociological study. It is often the vehicle of social reforms and social reorganisation.
6. A background knowledge of sociology is very useful for lawmakers to know the formal and informal laws of the country.
7. Sociology will improve international understanding and peace by evaluating the social cost of war and causes of social tension between nations.
8. Sociology is useful as a teaching subject. By desseminating knowledge about society, socialised thinking will emerge, socialised behaviour and new social order will be evolved. A knowledge of social forces is necessary for senior administrators (e.g. IAS cadre). Sociology can be taken up also as a full time profession.
9. Sociology has changed our outlook on crime and punishment. The criminals are no longer treated as degenerated beasts. They are now regarded as human beings suffering from mental deficiencies and efforts are accordingly made for their rehabilitation as useful members of society.
10. Tribal welfare—studies conducted by sociologists regarding tribal society and problems have helped many governments in undertaking various social welfare measures for tribals.

Uses of Sociology in Nursing

Medical Sociology

Medical sociology deals with medicine in modern society. Public health problems like epidemics, coronary heart diseases, hypertension, diabetes and intestinal disorders are caused largely by social factors of stress and the strain due to the fast modern life. Medical sociology is extremely useful for the entire health services. Sociologists examine diseases in their social settings, in the life of the community as well as the bedside and in the laboratory for they all have their social causes as well as individual causes. Prevention depends largely on dealing with the social causes. Doctor-patient and nurse-patient relationships, medical education and training, hospital administration, etc. are also studied in medical sociology.

Sociology is important to nursing in the following ways:

1. It will help the nurse to know the social life of the patients. The social environment plays an important part in the causation of health and disease. These factors include the cultural values, customs, beliefs, attitudes, morals, religion, education, standard of living, community life, availability of health services, social and political organisation. A harmonious social environment enables health, whereas maladjustment may not only cause illness but also deprive him of taking adequate action against it.
2. Sociology will enable her to know the distinctive culture of each patient. In a vast subcontinent like India with a variety of religions, castes, tribes and communities, it is essential to know the culture of each patient. This knowledge is necessary before attempting treatment to make medical and nursing services more effective. For this, an understanding of the subject of sociology is essential.
3. A knowledge of sociology will help the nurse to adjust herself with the situation in the hospital organisation and administration as this will influence the probable outcomes of the actions planned. The nurse must understand how personal goals, values, attitudes and emotional states of doctors and nurses build into life patterns of adjustments and how they influence the doctor-nurse relationships in the hospital context.
4. Nurses working in a community will realise that community is a population made up of several groups of people living in a certain area. Man is a social being and cannot live without the other human beings. Sociology is the study of society and social relations of how people react to one another. In sociology, we study man's picture of today's and tomorrow's society to find a way to a better life for all. Medical sociology will enable the nurse to:

a. Recognise the significance of social forces in health,
b. Understand and appreciate the need to deal with such social processes as health values and motivation, and
c. Organise and administer public health programmes as per motivational needs.

QUESTIONS

1. What is sociology? Explain the importance of study of sociology.
2. Explain the nature and scope of sociology with reference to nursing.
3. "Sociology is the science of society"—Discuss.
4. Sociology is of great 'practical utility'. Explain the role of nurses in society.
5. Mention any two differences between sociology and social psychology.
6. Who is the father of Sociology? Name any two Indian sociologists of repute.

18 Culture and Community Health

Culture is defined as the training and refinement of mind, taste and manners. Man is a product of his cultural environment. Culture is the product of human society and is handed down from one generation to the next. In general, culture stands for the mode of living, religion and law. It acts through tradition. Man picks up the culture of his society.

Culture influences health behaviour and health programmes of the population in the following areas:

1. Outlook on health and diseases.
2. Nutrition.
3. Mother and child health.
4. Women's health.
5. Personal hygiene.
6. Environmental sanitation.

Outlook on Health and Diseases

Health beliefs and practices are part of every culture. Ancient as well as many modern people consider disease is due to the wrath of supernatural powers. Sickness is considered as misfortune. In India, smallpox was considered to be due to the anger of goddess Sitala Devi. Diseases such as tuberculosis, leprosy and venereal diseases are considered punishment from supernatural powers for the past sins of the individual. People have great faith in *Hakims* and *Vaids*.

Nutrition

The food habits of people are a cultural heritage. Hindus do not eat meat. In Hindu society, vegetarianism is given a place of honour. Muslims and Jews do not eat pork. Jains do not eat curds. Horse meat is eaten in Europe but not in the United States. Some people regard cow's milk with a lot of prejudice. Many people do not take a particular food because they do not like its colour or smell. Some food fads and faulty food habits are listed below:

a. *Hot foods*: Meat, eggs, legumes and oil seeds increase heat production in the body and cause boils in the body.
b. *Cold foods:* Fruits, onions and curds decrease heat production in the body and cause cold and sore throat.
c. *Pica:* Eating clay by pregnant women helps in the normal development of the baby in the womb.
d. Garlic increases milk production in lactating women.
e. Papaya fruit and pineapple produces abortion in pregnant women.
f. Raw cucumber without salt is poisonous.
g. Vegetables, oils and fats are not fattening.
h. Drinking too much water is fattening.
i. Adults need no milk. (Wrong).

These believes have no scientific basis.

Practices Adversely Affecting Mother and Child Health

Certain foods such as eggs, meat and fish are forbidden during pregnancy in certain communities. In some parts of India, the child is not breastfed during the first three days after birth because they think that colostrum is harmful to the baby. Application of cowdung to the cut end of the umbilical cord is another bad custom, responsible for tetanus in the newborn. Branding of the skin and administration of castor oil are equally bad customs.

Women's Health

Cultural practices influencing contraceptive behaviour with reference to women's health:

a. Early marriage of girls expand the reproductive period of the girl child affecting her health, physical and mental maturity.
b. Preference for a male child prevents contraceptive practice of spacing which helps to regain the health of the mother and

provide her with free time with the elder child.

c. Low status of women—Women are deprived of basic nutritional food, shelter, clothing, education, freedom of speech, selection of mate, decision making, etc.
d. In many Indian communities, there is sex distinction in food habits too. In families, male members are fed first and then whatever is left is consumed by the female members of the house. This applies even to children. Boys are given the choicest of foods and girls are forced to eat whatever is given. Due to this, women are more prone to health problems like anaemia and calcium deficiency.
e. Taboos in discussing sexual problems openly with the kith and kin. This leads to increase in sexually transmitted diseases (STDs) and related health problems which further aggravate problems of modern family.

Personal Hygiene

Indians are very particular about their personal hygiene. Bathing is a daily routine with most Indians. The custom of applying oil before bath is a good Indian custom. Eating pan smeared with lime or without tobacco is a common social custom. Smoking hukka is another social custom in North India. Not wearing footwear transmits hookworm disease.

Environmental Health

The bulk of the rural population use the fields for defecation resulting in water and soil pollution and growth of flies. Pollution of water supplies is very common as people wash and bathe near water sources. Some rivers are considered 'holy' and people go on pilgrimage to have a dip in such rivers. They drink raw water which is responsible for outbreak of cholera and gastroenteritis.

Ecology and Aetiology of Diseases

Sociologists examine diseases in their social settings in the life of the community as well as by the bedside because diseases have both social and individual causes. Prevention depends largely on dealing with the social causes.

1. Coal miners develop black lung disease. Men working with asbestos develop lung cancer and those working with polyvinyl chloride (PVC) plastics develop liver cancer. Sociologists have established a close relationship between psychosomatic diseases like coronary diseases, cancer, peptic ulcer and some mental diseases and stress.
2. Variation in attitudes and behaviour affects health and illness.
3. Many diseases, while selecting their victims, differentiate such social variables as age, sex, socioeconomic status, racial ethnic group identity, education and occupation.

In developing countries, incidence of infant mortality and infectious diseases like malaria, tuberculosis, dysentery, cholera, typhoid and chickenpox is higher. In advanced countries, where people's life expectancy is high, a higher incidence of cancer, heart diseases, rheumatism as well as mental disorders are more common. Genetic factors cannot account for these. The main biological causes of ill health of people in underdeveloped countries is their inferior nutrition, living conditions and inadequate health services. In the 19th century, the present advanced countries too had infant mortality and incidence of infectious diseases, similar to the people in backward countries today. That was also due to similar conditions like malnutrition, overcrowding, impure water and poor sanitation. Economic development and rapid advances in public health services soon improved their conditions. It reduced the incidence of preventable misery, suffering and loss of life caused by major infections in those countries.

QUESTIONS

1. Define culture. Mention any one feature of culture.
2. Explain how social features influence health and illness.
3. Mention any two specific beliefs in Indian culture which have beneficial health effects.
4. Mention any two religions practices which have adverse effects on health and family welfare .

19 The Individual: Growth and Development

GROWTH

Growth refers to an increase in physical size of the whole body or any of it's parts. Growth is because of cell division and the synthesis of proteins. It causes a quantitative change in the child's body. It can be measured in Cms and Kgs. The process of growth covers nearly a third of human lifespan.

DEVELOPMENT

Development refers to a progression in skill and capacity to function. It causes qualitative changes in the child's functioning.

Growth and development are so closely interrelated that when growth in any stage is slow or rapid, the development also is affected in the same way.

The period of growth and development extends throughout the lifecycle. Principal changes occur during the period from conception to the end of adolescence.

NURSE'S RESPONSIBILITY

A knowledge of growth and development is important to the nurse for the following reasons:

1. To know what to expect of a particular child at any given age.
2. To plan for nursing management of each child.
3. To better understand the reason for particular conditions and illnesses that occur in various age groups.
4. To teach parents to observe and to use their knowledge, so that they may help their children achieve optimum growth and development.

Harmful Prenatal Environment

Healthy, well nourished mothers experience throughout their pregnancies fewer complications such as anaemia, abortion and premature delivery. The foetus may suffer from nutritional deficiencies when the mother's diet is insufficient in quality and quantity. Mother's diabetes mellitus may affect the foetus. Rubella (German measles) during the first trimester of pregnancy may cause abnormal development of the foetus.

Behaviour Problems in Children

Every child has certain basic emotional needs which ought to be satisfied to ensure his optimal development as an emotionally mature individual.

According to United Nations Declaration on the Right of the child: (1) Every child has the right to affection, love and understanding. The child is dependant on parents, who should ensure for him, (2) A sense of belonging and security. He should be able to trust them. They should accept him as an individual in his own right and should give him, (3) An increasing independence within the limitations imposed by the society. Although the child seeks autonomy, he should be under some discipline, so that he can conform to the social and cultural norms, (4) The milieu of the child should promote confidence and self-respect, (5) Opportunities should be made available for play, activity and recreation, (6) He should be able to take pride in his achievements, (7) Every child wishes to model himself after his parents and therefore he should have, and (8) Adequate social and emotional interactions with parents.

Parent-child Maladjustment

Active support and cooperation of parents are essential for adequate management of behavioural problems in their children. Parental attitudes which lead to maladjustment are:

a. *Rejection:* Birth of an unwanted child, or a child of the sex other than the desired sex, or of disputed paternity may lead to rejection. The child easily perceives the lack of warmth in the parent's attitude.
b. *Overdominance* by the parent.
c. *Overprotection:* An overprotective parent may prevent the child develop his sense of independence and autonomy.
d. *Unrealistic expectations:* The parents may push the child to achieve scholastic goals, much beyond his level of competence. A conflict between the child's achievements and parent's aspirations increases the stress.
e. Inconsistent discipline.
f. Unhealthy criticism and unfavourable comparisons.
g. Broken home or parental discord.
h. *Sibling rivalry:* With the birth of a younger sibling, the older child may be deprived of love and security which can lead to behavioural disturbances. To avoid such situations, the older child should be involved in the care of the younger sibling under parental watch.

Problems of Adjustment in the School

A poor child, when placed in an expensive school, patronized by richer children may find it impossible to bridge the gap. He may develop an inferiority complex and hate his parents for their inability to provide him with a similar environment as his rich peers. This results in the child's maladjustment with his peers and teachers.

Problems of Adolescence

They include:
1. Juvenile delinquency.
2. Scholastic underachievement.
3. Learning disabilities.

Juvenile Delinquency

A child or adolescent is considered juvenile delinquent when he indulges in unlawful activities habitually and repeatedly. Children between age seven and eighteen for boys and girls come under the purview of Juvenile Justice Act of 1986. Causes of juvenile delinquency, according to Healy and Bronner are: (1) Bad company, (2) Adolescent instability and impulses, (3) Early sex experience, (4) Mental conflicts, (5) Extreme social suggestivity, (6) Love of adventures, (7) Motion picture, (8) School dissatisfaction, (9) Poor recreation, (10) Street life, (11) Vocational dissatisfaction, (12) Sudden impulses, and (13) Physical conditions of all sorts. For further details turn to chapter 26, Social Problems (delinquency) page 200.

EFFECT OF ENVIRONMENT ON CHILDHOOD, ADOLESCENCE, ADULTHOOD AND OLD AGE

Individuals differ from each other because they reveal different personalities. These differences are due to interaction of two powerful factors—Heredity and environment.

Heredity refers to the biological process of transmission of certain biological and psychological characteristics from parents to their children through genes.

Environment is anything immediately surrounding an organism and exert a direct influence on it. The role of the environment is so great that it can affect our society and our behaviour.

Children of the same heredity (identical twins) are placed under different environment and observed. The differences in their behaviour are due to changes in the environment.

The nature (heredity)-nature (environment) controversy is regarding the relative importance of heredity and environment in human development. But sociologists are now agreed that our development is not due to heredity alone or environment alone but due to both equally. Heredity provides our potential for development which will be realised by a favourable environment. No more do we say heredity or environment but heredity and environment. They are interdependent forces.

However, it is still not possible to say with certainty what behaviour traits are influenced by heredity/environment. Heredity factors appear to be more prominent in the following areas: Reflex and instinctive behaviour, blood type, finger prints, eye colour, colour and texture of hair and skin, chromosomal abnormalities and defective genes, schizophrenia, haemophilia, tuberculosis and some cancers.

Environmental factors influence human interests, attitudes, aptitudes, habits, temperament, social and cultural norms as well as manners and etiquette. Environmental effects are maximum in the earlier years of human life when we are most impressionable.

Effect of Environment

Childhood

The development task during infancy is trust versus mistrust. The infant learns slowly that when he is cold, wet or hungry, there is the mother (or mother substitute) who will redress it with loving care. If the child is given affection and all his needs are met, the child will feel that the world is safe and dependable. The child will identify his mother and other members of his family who are always with him. Trust is formed because of consistency, continuity and sameness of the child's experience. On the other hand, if the child is neglected and the treatment given by the adults is inconsistent, the outcome will be mistrust and stranger anxiety.

When an infant does not receive warm and loving care, or is isolated from others or from his natural environment, the condition is called need deprivation. Deprivation has far reaching consequences on the emotional and intellectual development of the child.

Nurse and the Child

An infant is in the need of tender loving care both at home and in the hospital. Many hospitals have nurseries for nurse care for the infant for the duration of its stay in the hospital. The nurse should plan to give as much personal attention as possible, such as handling, cuddling, holding and loving the infant in her care.

During early childhood, the child may be weaned when nursing becomes painful to the mother. The child learns that it cannot entirely depend on his mother for all his needs and that he has to take some degree of care himself. The child learns to control elimination of waste and do things for himself. The child needs encouragement to do new things. If the child is respected as an individual, the child will develop a sense of autonomy, otherwise feeling of shame and doubt about himself will be developed.

During the middle and late childhood, the child compares himself with others and will feel productive and industrious, if he is successful with his peers. Child feels inferior if he fails to meet the social expectations of his parents and for the first time, those outside his home (in the school).

Keeping a good relationship with growing children will be quite a challenge to the nurse. The child will be selfcentred and may not cooperate. The nurse must be patient with children; use of force and violence must be scrupulously avoided. An anxious child does not recover well. Therefore the nurse must give love, affection and care. The child's emotional needs must be taken care of and he should be encouraged to feel cheerful and independent.

Adolescence

The transition from childhood to adulthood is known as adolescence. Through physical, social and mental changes, the child must develop into adult life.

Adolescence is a period of stress and storm. Life is at disequilibrium and the adolescent suffers from identity crisis. Development task at this stage is to develop a sense of identity regarding occupational, familial and social roles. This requires a stable, loving home and wise and mature parents who understand the needs of their children and treat them as growing individuals. Soon the adolescent will free himself from his parents and look for his own identity as against role confusion. This state causes one to feel isolated, empty, anxious and indecisive. Adolescence comes to an end with adulthood. Helping adolescents to feel good about themselves will promote a good nurse-patient relationship.

Adulthood

The major development task of adulthood include selecting a life partner, establishing a home and accepting responsibility of the parent. Children cannot be effectively nurtured unless family has security. A successful parent also should be a good citizen and a participating member of a social group.

The adult patient may be desperate with secret fears and anxieties. It is desirable if the nurse tries to probe into the tense behaviour of adult patients.

Old Age

Old people have to adjust to reduced income and deteriorating health. Frequently friends and spouse die leading to loneliness. Besides physical weakness, there is general infirmity and mental deterioration. Memory is weak, power of adjustment poor. For some old people, life is futile and a burden. It is the society's responsibility to provide a suitable environment for old people to live in dignity and sense of order and meaning to life. They should not be made to feel that they are being neglected because of their incapacity to work and earn.

Generally old people become impatient and show irritability and willfulness. The nurse should realise that these are due to the normal deterioration process.

QUESTIONS

1. What are the two factors on which human behaviour is based?
2. What is heredity?
3. What are the essential characters inherited by all the human beings?
4. When does the environment affect man the most?
5. Describe the effect of environment on children.
6. Explain how does the environment affect man during his adolescence.
7. How does the environment affect man during the adulthood and old age.

20 Fundamental Rights and Fundamental Duties

The Right and Responsibilities of Individuals in Democratic Society

The constitution of India (in part III) has classified fundamental rights which are to act as limitations not only on the powers of the executive but also upon the powers of legislature. The fundamental rights as per part III of the constitution are:

1. Right to equality.
2. Right to particular freedoms.
3. Right against exploitation.
4. Right to freedom of religion.
5. Cultural and educational rights.
6. Right to constitutional remedies.

The rights falling under each of the six categories are as in Table 20.1. Right to free education for children upto 14 years has been incorporated with effect from 1st April 2010.

These rights are called fundamental rights because they are guaranteed by the constitution and cannot be taken away by an individual or group or even by the government. The purpose of these rights is to safeguard the liberty of the people. They act as safeguard against any abuse of power by the government.

Some fundamental rights are granted only to citizens of India: (a) Protection against discrimination on grounds only on religion, race, caste, sex or place of birth (Art 15), (b) Equality of opportunity in matters of public employment (Art 16), (c) Freedom of speech, assembly, association, movement, residence and profession (Art 19), (d) Cultural and educational rights of minorities (Art 30).

Some of the fundamental rights on the other hand are

Table 20.1: Fundamental rights

Right to equality	Right to freedom	Right against exploitation	Right to freedom of religion	Cultural and educational rights	Right to constitutional remedies
1. Equality before law and equal pro-traction before law (Art 14)	1. Freedom of speech and expression; assembly; association; movement; residence and settlement; ....[1] profession (Art 19)	1. Prohibition of traffic in human beings and forced labour (Art 23)	1. Freedom of conscience and free profession (Art 25)	1. Protection of language, script or culture of minorities (Art 29)	Remedies for enforcement of the fundamental rights conferred by this Part,—writs of habeas corpus, mandamus, prohibition, certiorari and quo warranto (Art 32)
2. Prohibition of discrimination on ground of religion, etc. (Art 15)	2. Protection in respect of conviction for offences (Art 20)	2. Prohibition of employment of children in hazardous employment (Art 24)	2. Freedom to manage religious affairs (Art 26)	2. Right of minorities to establish and administer educational institutions (Art 30)	
3. Equality of opportunity in employment (Art 16)	3. Protection of life and personal liberty (Art 21)		3. Freedom as to payment of taxes for promotion of any particular religion (Art 27)	3. Right of children between 7 to 14 years for free and compulsory education with effect from 1-4-2010)	
4. Abolition of untouchability (Art 17)	4. Protection against arrest and detention in certain cases (Art 22)		4. Freedom as to attendance at religious instruction in certain educational institutions (Art 28)		
5. Abolition of titles (Art 18)					

[1]Right to property omitted from Part III of the constitution, by the constitution (44th Amendment) Act, 1978.

available to any person on the soil of India—citizen or foreigner: (a) Equality before law and equal protection of laws (Art 14). (b) Protection in respect of conviction against ex post-facto laws, double punishment and self-incrimination (Art 20), (c) Protection of life and personal liberty against action without authority of law (Art 21), (d) Right against exploitation (Art 23), (e) Freedom of religion (Art 25), (f) Freedom as to payment of taxes for the promotion of any religion (Art 27), and (g) Freedom as to attendance of religious instruction or worship in state educational institutions.

Fundamental Duties

There are ten fundamental duties incorporated in the constitution which brings our constitution in line with the Universal Declaration of Human Rights and constitutions of Japan, China and Russia. These duties were added as Art 51A (Part IV A) of the constitution by the 42nd amendment Act 1976. Under this article it shall be the duty of every citizen of India:

1. To abide by the constitution and respect the national flag and national anthem.
2. To cherish and follow the noble ideals which inspired our national struggle for freedom.
3. To protect the sovereignity, unity and integrity of India.
4. To defend the country.
5. To promote the spirit of common brotherhood amongst all people of India.
6. To preserve the rich heritage of our composite culture.
7. To protect and improve the natural environment.
8. To develop the scientific temper and spirit of enquiry.
9. To safeguard public property.
10. To strive towards excellence in all spheres of individual and collective activity.

These duties are obligatory for every citizen, even though there is no provision in the constitution for direct enforcement of any of these duties nor any sanction for their violation. But they serve as a warning to reckless citizens against antisocial activities such

Table 20.2: Directive principles of state policy

Directives in the nature of ideals of the state	Directives shaping the policy of the states	Non-justiciable rights of citizens
1. The state shall strive to promote the welfare of the people by securing a social order permeated by social, economic and political justice [Art 38(1)]. to minimise inequality in income, status, facilities and opportunities, amongst individuals and groups [Art 38 (2)].	1. To establish economic democracy and justice by securing certain economic rights (to be enumerated in the next column)	1. Right to adequate means of livelihood [Art 39 (a)]
2. The state shall endeavour to secure just and human conditions of work, a living wage, a decent standard of living and social and cultural opportunities for all workers (Art 43).	2. To secure a uniform civil code for the citizens (Art 44).	2. Right of both sexes to euqal pay for equal work [Art 39 (d)]
3. The state shall endeavour to raise the level of nutrition and standard for living and to improve public health (Art 47).	3. To provide free and compulsory primary education (Art 45)	3. Right against economic expolitation [Art 39 (e)-(f)]
4. The state shall direct its policy towards securing quitable distribution of the material resources of the community and prevention of concentration of wealth and means of production [Art 39 (b)-(c)].	4. To prohibit consumption of liquor and intoxicating drugs except for medical purposes (Art 47)	4. *Right of children and the young to be proected against exploitation and to opportunities for healthy development, consonant with freedom and dignity [Art 39 (f)]*[2]
5. The state shall endeavour to promote international peace and amity (Art 51)	5. To develop cottage industries (Art 43)	5. Right to equal opportunity for justice and free legal aid (Art 39A)[2]
	6. To organise agriculture and animal husbandry on modern line (Art 48)	6. Right to work (Art 41)

Contd...

Contd...

	7. To prevent slaughter of useful cattle, i.e. cows, calves, and other milch and draught cattle (Art 48)	7. Right to public assistance in case of unemployment, old age, sickness and other cases of undeserved want (Art 41).
	8. To organise village panchayats as units of self-government (Art 40)	8. *Right to humane conditions of work and maternity relief (Art 42)*
	9. To promote educational and economic interests of weaker sections and to protect them from social injustice (Art 46)	9. Right to a living wage and conditions of work ensuring decent standard of life for workers (Art 43)
	10. To protect and improve the environment and to safeguard forests and wild life (Art 48A)[2]	10. *Right of workers to participate in management of industries (Art 43A)*[2]
	11. To protect and maintain places of historic or artistic interest (Art 49).	11. Right of children to free and compulsory education (Art 45)
	12. To separate the judiciary from the executive (Art 50)	

1. Added by the 44th Amendment Act, 1978
2. Added by the 42nd Amendment Act, 1976

as burning of the constitution, destroying public property and the like.

The legal utility of the fundamental duties is similar to the directive principles of our constitution given in Table 20.2. While the directives are addressed to the state without any legal sanction, the duties are addressed to the citizen without any legal sanction for their violation. The citizen is to be his own judge while exercising and enforcing his fundamental duties—remembering that he owes the duties specified in Art 51 (A) to the state—that if he does not care for the duties he does not deserve the rights. For example, if he burns the constitution, in violation of his duty in Art 51 (A), he cannot assert that the meeting at which he brunt the constitution by way of demonstration against the government, be protected by the freedom of expression or assembly guaranteed by Art 19.

QUESTIONS

1. What are the rights of an Indian Citizen?
2. What are the responsibilities of an individual in a democratic society?

21 The Family

Family is one of the oldest institutions of the world. It is found even in the most primitive of human societies. There is no society in the world where family is not found. Man's social life begins with the family. Family is a primary group which is the centre of most of our life activities. It gives shape to our personality and provides us inspiration. Our success or failure in life, to certain extent, depends on the family.

Family fulfils the basic needs of the society. It is the cradle of civilisation of the child. It is the first social environment to which a child is exposed. It is where health habits are learned by the child.

Meaning of the Term "Family"

The word "family" has been taken over from the Latin word "*Famulus*" which means a servant. In Roman law, the word denoted a group of producers and slaves and other servants as well as members connected by common descent or marriage. Thus originally family consisted of a man and woman with a child or children and servants. The meaning of family can be explained by the following definitions.

Definitions of Family

1. *MF Nimkoff:* "Family is more or less a durable association of husband and wife with or without child or of a man or woman alone, with children."
2. *Burgess and Lecke:* "Family is a group of persons united by ties of marriage, blood or adoption constituting a single household interacting and inter-communicating with each other in their

respective social roles of husband and wife, father and mother, son and daughter, brother and sister, creating a common culture."

3. *Eliot and Merrill:* Family is "the biological social unit composed of husband, wife and children".
4. *MacIver:* Family is "a group defined by relationship sufficiently precise and enduring to provide for the procreation and upbringing of children."

General Characteristics of a Family

Out of these definitions, the following characteristics of a family may be derived:

1. *A mating relationship:* A family comes into existence when a man and a woman establish a mating relationship between them.
2. *Selection of mates:* Wife or husband may be selected by parents or by elders or the choice may be left to the wishes of the individuals themselves. Various rules govern this selection.
3. *A form of marriage:* The mating relationship is established through the institution of marriage. Marriage is an institutional arrangement made by the society according to which individuals establish marital relationships among themselves. Marriage may assume any one of the forms—monogamy, polygamy, polyandry or group marriage.
4. *A system of nomenclature or name:* Every family is known or recognised by a distinctive name.
5. *A way of tracing the descent:* Every family has its own mode of tracing the descent. Descent refers to the social recognition of biological relationship between individuals. Descent may be traced through the male line (patrilineal descent), or through the female line (matrilineal descent) or through both the lines (Bilateral descent).
6. *A common residence:* A family needs a home or household for its living.
7. *An economic provision:* Family provides for the satisfaction of the economic needs of its members.

Functions of the Family

Family is the nucleus of all social groups because of the importance of its functions. MacIver classifies the function of the family into:
1. Essential or primary and
2. Non-essential or secondary functions.

Essential Functions (Necessary for the Continued Existence of the Society Itself)

1. *Stable satisfaction of sex:* The first essential function of the family is sex gratification. Generally societies accept and approve sexual relationship between husband and wife as legitimate. Family is designed to provide a life long. partnership to the spouses. This avoides uncertainty and sex rivalry. Family also helps to develop sexual harmony and better personality adjustments.
2. *The reproductive function:* Every society depends primarily on the family for the production of children.
3. *Provision of a home:* Family provides home for its members. The desire for home is strongly felt in man and women. Irrespective of their actual place of birth (hospitals/nursing homes) children are nurtured and sustained at home. Parents who work outside are dependent on their home for comfort, protection and peace. Home still remains and will remain the sweet place to seek refuge in.
4. *Socialisation function:* Socialisation is the process whereby one internalises the norms of one's group, so that a distinct self-emerges, unique to the individual. The family indoctrinates the child with values, morals, beliefs and ideals of the society. It prepares its children for participation in a larger world. Family provides the models for the child to imitate. Indeed family is an agent of socialisation.
5. *Affectional function:* Family provides the mental or emotional satisfaction and security for its members. It provides the most intimate and dearest relationship for all its members. The individual first experiences love in his parental family as parents

and siblings offer him sympathy and affection. Lack of affection actually damages an infants ability to thrive. A person who has not received love and affection during childhood cannot be happy in adult life.

6. *The status function:* Family is the source of our social identification. Various statuses are initially ascribed by our families. Our class status, residential status, religious status, educational status, etc. are conferred on us by our families.
7. *Protective function:* Family offers some degree of physical, economic and psychological protection to its members. In many societies any attack on any of its members is considered as an attack on the family itself.

Secondary Functions of Family

1. *Economic functions:* The family fulfils the economic needs of its members. This has been the traditional function of the family. Previously family was an economic unit, goods were produced in the family. Now the economic role of modern family is considerably modified. The process of industrialisation has affected the family. The family members do not work together at home. The centre of production has moved from home to the factory.
2. *Educational function:* The family provides the basis for the child's formal learning. In spite of great changes, the family still provides the child his basic training in the social attitudes and habits. When the child grows up he learns to manage the situations outside the home and family in the same manner he learned how to get along with the members of his family earlier. He extents his interests to other groups.
3. *Religious functions:* Family is the centre for the religious training of the children. The religious values, moral precepts and worshiping God, etc. are taught in the family. The family lays down the moral standards that are to guide the children throughout their lives. The family meets the spiritual needs of its members. It is through the family that the religious inheritance is passed on to the next generation.

Health Functions of the Family

In addition to the above, a basic family function is to protect the health of the family members and to provide supportive nurturing care during period of illness. In an earlier era, when hospitals were rare, bedridden patients were treated at their homes. It is within the family that members of the family develop their concept of health habits. The family as a social unit, develops a system of values, beliefs and attitudes about health and illness behaviours of its members. It is through family, that members learn the belief and practices of the larger society concerning health and illness. Family also transmits health related cultural traits to next generations.

The health related functions and tasks of family are:

1. Provision of adequate food, shelter and clothing.
2. Maintenance of health supporting physical environment at home.
3. Maintenance of health supporing psychological environment.
4. Provision of resources for maintenance of personal hygiene.
5. Health education.
6. Promotion of health by nutrition and exercise.
7. Recognition of health disruption.
8. Health and illness decision making.
9. First aid.
10. Seeking health care, illness care and dental care.
11. Supervision of medication.
12. Provision for meeting spiritual needs.
13. Rehabilitation care.
14. Interaction with community health personnel.

FAMILY AS A UNIT OF COMMUNITY HEALTH SERVICE

Family as a social institution is the basic unit of health services. It is the focal point of health care and the right place for integrating, preventive, promotive and curative services. The family system is a baisc unit within which the health behaviour including health values, health habits and health risk perceptions are developed, organised and performed. The interrelationship between health, health behaviour and the family is a highly dynamic one in which each may have a dramatic effect on others.

Definition of Family Health

Family health is the continuing ability of the family to meet defined functions in the interaction with other social, political, economic and health systems.

Determinants of Family Health

The external environment includes climate, terrain, air, safe water supply, biological environment (insects, rodents) and man made physical environment, i.e. location, construction of house surroundings, etc. The internal environment of the family includes its size, structure, type of members, their relationships, biological characteristics, cultural patterns and values.

Family Health and Community Health Nurse

A thorough knowledge of the above factors obtaining in her particular area, is very essential for the community health nurse to assess the health-illness situations that affect family health. She identifies the key issues and plays the multiple role such as counsellor, teacher, coordinator, facilitator, case finder, supervisor and refer to monitor the health and welfare of families in her particular area.

Basic Needs of the Family

1. *Physical:* Food, shelter, clothing, safe physical environment (e.g. safe drinking water, proper disposal of waste).
2. *Biological:* Freedom from communicable diseases, control of pests, insects and vectors, control of rodents, planned parenthood.
3. *Psychological needs:* A happy home, a safe working environment, freedom from poverty, adequate medical care, social security for all its members, care of special groups— mothers and children, aged, handicapped, and women.

Types or Forms of Family

On the basis of the nature of residence, descent, succession and authority structure, families can be classified into:
1. Matrilineal family
2. Patriarchal family.

FAMILY IN INDIA

The family in India is based on patrilenial descent. Children are identified by name and allegiance with the father's family.

Property is passed on from one generation to the next within the family.

Joint Family

"A joint family is a group of people who generally live under one roof, who eat food cooked at one heath, who hold property in common and who participate in common worship and are related to each other as some particular type of kindred" —
—Smt Iravathi Karve.

Nuclear family	Joint family
It is the outcome of modern influences.	It is made up of a number of nuclear families, which are all related. All of them live in a common house.
This kind of family consists of husband, wife and their offsprings. More in urban India.	All the blood relations like grand-parents, parents, grandchildren uncles, aunts and their children and other relations live together. Such families are found in rural India.
The advantage is that they have individual freedom but no social or economical security during calamities.	But with the advent of inodernism and urban influence, joint family is slowly disappearing.

Advantages of Joint Family

1. Division of labour
2. Advantageous for agricultural economy
3. Provides minimum existence
4. Encourages social virtues

5. Insurance against hard times.
6. More leisure—all for each and each for all
7. Socialistic pattern—contribution according to capacity but receiving as per each person's need.

Disadvantages of Joint Family

1. Encourages idleness
2. Hinders full development
3. Leads to quarrels
4. Miserable condition of women
5. No privacy
6. Lower living standards
7. Perpetuates orthodoxy by discouraging progressive outlook
8. Leads to litigation.

RECENT TRENDS IN MODERN INDIAN FAMILY OR DISINTEGRATION OF JOINT FAMILY

1. *Industrialisation:* Joint family system is most suited to agricultural function. Industrial revolution has affected the economic functions of the family with the birth of many factories. Workers from villages are moving to the cities breaking the joint families. Industrialisation and urbanisation go together. Cities are growing in size and in number. Family is cut to size.
2. *Decline of agriculture and cottage industries:* The joint family system flourished in India when agriculture and village industries were at their best. Today, the village craftsmen cannot compete with goods produced by mechanised factories. With the decline in cottage industries, the craftsmen migrate to the cities for employment. Due to pressure on land, the agricultural workers are also compelled to seek work in cities.
3. *Impact of the West:* India today is greatly influenced by the social outlook by Western thought and democratic ideologies. Democracy assures quality and provides equality for all. Women now play not only domestic roles but also economic and political roles. The woman has now become an equal

earning member. The economic independance has increased her status and affected her attitude. Individualism has made deep inroads into Indian society.

4. *Decline of mores and religious beliefs:* Morality and religion are slowly losing ground. Family members have become more secular in their outlook. Religious functions of the family have decreased. Individualism and romantic love are widespread. They have destroyed the authority of family over the individual members.
5. *Improved communication and transport facilities:* As the means of communication and transport facilities are improved, it is no longer necessary for men to stay with the family and carry on the family occupation. Now they go to cities.
6. *New social legislations:* The joint family system has been influenced by social legislation like the Civil Marriage Act 1872, the Hindu Marriage Act 1956 and the Hindu Succession Act 1956. The Civil Marriage Act enables adult boys and girls to get married even against the wishes of their parents. It has encouraged free choice of mates. Marriage has become also easily dissolvable as it is entered by mutual consent of partners. Marriage has become more and more a civil contract.
7. *Generation gap:* Interpersonal conflicts in the family is on the increase. An unusual amounts of conflicts between parents and their adolescent children are taking place. Decline of birth rate is adversely affecting the joint family. Divorce, desertion and separation are quite common.

CONCLUSION

All these are symptoms and signs of modern family, coping itself with the stress and strain of modern era. The family is merely seeking to adapt itself to changed conditions.

The Family Cycle

Due to modern influences, the joint families are breaking up giving place to nuclear families. When the children in the nuclear family grow up and marry, a joint family is again created which in turn break up into nuclear families and the process is repeated over and over again. This process is called the life-cycle of a family. It emphasizes the importance of family members and basic needs of the family.

The infant begins life well protected but soon faces many uncompromising demands from the parents, siblings and relatives. Each person is different and since rights and duties differ in each family, there are variations in the interaction between members in each family.

Mother and her infant establish close emotional relationship to each other early in the childhood. The world of the child soon expands and spreads to include other members of the family. The daughter identifies herself with the mother and son with his father and grow up to adulthood. Both parents establish love ties with the children and gradually develop a spirit of independence in them.

The society in which the child grows up is different from the society in which the parents grew up. The parent takes his childhood experiences as a guide to teach his children but this would not suit the present day children. This is popularly known as the "generation gap". Parents should take note of this problem and try to change their attitude towards their children. Otherwise conflicts will arise alienating the children from the parents.

QUESTIONS

1. What is the most important unit (group) of human society? How is it made of?
2. Define marriage. Describe its functions and purposes.
3. Give a brief account of the major forms of marriage.
4. What is a family, what are its main characteristics?
5. Explain the social and functional importance of family.
6. What are the functions of family? Explain.
7. Explain the family's role in the health of the children.
8. Explain the problems of modern family.
9. Describe any six characteristics of Joint Hindu family.
10. Describe any six disadvantages of joint family.

11. What factors have caused changes in the joint family system?
12. Is joint family relevant to the Indian social situation at present? Discuss.
13. Is the Hindu joint family disintegrating? Substantiate your answer with proper examples.
14. What are the different types of family?
15. What are the benefits of a joint family?
16. Bring the functions of modern family.
17. What is family? Describe the types and functions of family and the changes occurred in the modern family.

22 Family Life Education

Family life education refers to those educational concepts and experiences that influence attitudes towards family living, personal relationships and sexual development.

Family life education includes a study of awareness, understanding of others, of sexuality, marriage and parenthood, so that this knowledge will contribute to the individual ability to cope both with social changes and with relationships in society as a citizen, spouse and parent.

Specific objectives of family life education

Components	***Objectives***
1. Concepts of family types and purposes	a. To identify the historical functions of a family and its different structures b. To define the term family life education c. To identify various types of facilities d. To identify various types of families
2. Family relationship and responsibility	a. To identify various aspects of relationships of various members of family b. To define the responsibilities and functions of each member

Married life is not easy. It never was Marriage is one of the most stressful relationships between a man and a woman, but like democracy, the best available. Marriages often fail not because of the problems encountered but because of the inadequacy of preparations involved. There would be a lot more contentment in married life, if the couple had entered the marriage not with their heads in the clouds but with their feet firmly on the ground, that is without unreasonable hopes, expectations and demands. Disappoints in marriage is the difference between what one expects and what one actually gets. A generally happy marriage is the result of years of patient and persistent effort, both before and after the marriage.

On the Threshold of Marriage

The young couple, on the threshold of marriage feel the need to know more about and plan better for the way of life they are about to start. They will not be satisfied by vague assurances that everything will be alright in due course. They will want to know more. They have every right to know what is necessary to make their marriage successful and happy. Young people planning marriage need helpful guidance to create harmonious partnership which is basic to a successful marriage.

Development of such education would make the individual more aware of his/her responsibilities and consequences of his/her sexual behaviour.

Lack of proper sex education can lead to:

1. Crimes of eve teasing, molesting, rape and child assault.
2. Drug abuse, STDs and HIV/AIDS.
3. Body dysfunction like impotency, frigidity, premature ejaculation, etc.
4. Marital maladjustment leading to divorce and single parenthood.

Community health nurses of today have a significant role in effectively carrying out the sex education programmes in schools and colleges as also other groups in the community.

In India progress in this direction has been very slow as any discusson on matters of sex is still considered taboo by most of our population. But sex education has to be introduced urgently in our schools and colleges to help the youth to lead a healthy life.

This will make them responsible parents and may be an answer to India's population explosion.

Sex education should form an integral part of the school syllabus. Whenever, students have doubts about sex or AIDS, the questions have to be addressed. Sex education must not only comprise information about the act itself. It must educate the student on sexuality, developing life skills, AIDS, STD and myths; otherwise difficult questions tend to be answered by "do it yourself method".

Preparative Course for Marriage

Young people should be made to realise the responsibilities of marriage and duties of family life by attending a counselling course of two or three weeks' duration with psychologists, doctors practising lawers and religious teachers as resource persons. The course must cover subjects like inherited diseases, sex education, planned parenthood, STDs, legal conditions of a valid marriage, rights and responsibilities of the partners, Indian marriage as a sacrement, separation and divorce, property rights and other relevant aspects.

Today a wife and mother is expected to be an inspiring companion to her husband, proficient in the care of children, able in managing the family budget, good in home management and provide tasty and nutritions food to all family members and guests. Similarly a husband and father is expected to be the provider for his wife and children, protector of home and provider of domestic harmony based on mutual respect. Both should have good emotional qualities like patience, kindness, understanding, prudence, tolerance, fortitude and loyality. Thus, married life is more than a fulltime job demanding a high sense of duty and adequate preparation.

The modern young woman's increased personal and social maturity may cause certain adjustment problems in marriage. Traditionally, the wife was completely subordinate to her husband. Today, there is growing tendency towards equal authority and more companionship between the couple.

However, the main role of the wife will continue to be that of home making and taking care of the children. The man will remain the breadwinner and protector. At the same time, they will have to learn to be equal partners in running a home and sharing everything together.

Sex Education

Sex education in schools and colleges is necessary to prepare adolescent boys and girls to face the realities of life.

Aims of Sex Education

1. To have the correct knowledge about sex and sexuality.
2. To understand and be comfortable with ones own sexuality so as to be able to handle adolescent changes both physical and emotional.
3. To establish such social relationship with individuals of the same as well as the opposite sex with mutual respect and concern.
4. As the first step towards a happy and healthy married life in future.

QUESTIONS

1. Describe the family's role in the health of the children.
2. Describe the advantages of family life education.
3. Explain why family planning is necessary in a country like India.

23 Social Groups

"Man is a social animal" said Aristotle long ago. No normal man lives alone. Individual needs the group often and a person belongs to several different groups at one time to meet different needs. A group may be of large number or only two or three persons.

Social group is any collection of persons who share some common interest and reason for being together. Some groups are formed naturally; others are organised for a particular purpose.

Characteristics of Groups

1. Collection of individuals
2. Interaction among members
3. Group unity and solidarity
4. Group interests
5. Group norms
6. Size
7. Dynamic aspects of groups
8. Stability
9. Influence on personality.

Classification of Social Groups

Groups are classified into different types on the basis of size, nature of interaction, group interest, age, sex, class, caste, nationality, race and religion.

Primary and Secondary Groups

The classification of social groups into "primary" and secondary has become very popular today. American social psychologist CH

Cooley has introduced the term "primary group" in his book "social organisation" Primary groups such as family, small and long-lasting has close contact and face to face relationship. Secondary group is a collection of individuals with some common interests and aims—Membership is voluntary and relationship formal (Table 23.1).

Table 23.1: Comparison between primary and secondary groups

Primary group	**Secondary group**	
1. Meaning	Groups which are characterised by face to face relations, mutual aid and companionships, e.g. family, neighbourhood community, children's play-group, local brotherhood.	Groups which provide experience, but lacking in intimacy, e.g. political parties, trade unions, religious associations, the state, corporation, factory, rotary club.
2. Nature of social relations	Social relations are face to face, direct, intimate personal, non-contractual, nonspecialised, non-partisan and noneconomic in character.	Social relations are indirect, impersonal, non-intimate, contractual, specialised, partisan and more economic in nature.
3. Size	Primary groups are smaller in size (2 to 50). They are localised or limited to a definite area.	Relatively bigger in size They are not necessarily restricted to a small area.
4. Social proximity	Groups are confined to a small geographic area.	Groups are not characte-rised by a physical area.
5. Comm-unication	Since members stay together, communication is not only direct but also quick and effective.	Since members are spread over a vast area, direct communication is difficult. It is mostly indirect in nature.
6. Group interests	Interests of members are not specific but general everyone is interested in the welfare of everyone else.	Interests of members are specific, hence, groups are called special interest groups.

Contd...

Contd...

7. Nature of coopera-tion	Cooperation is direct, members work together, play together, enjoy together and in times of crisis struggle together. Cooperation is natural and spontaneous.	Cooperation is mostly indirect cooperation, is an intended act to serve a particular need. It is limi ted to that purpose only. It is not spontaneous but deliberate and cultivated.
8. Group structure	Very informal. Members are not very particular about their right, power, stature or prestige. No formal and detailed rules are drafted as guidelines.	Group structure is formal. The group is regulated by a set of formal rules. Statutes and roles. Rights and powers of members are well defined. The organisation of the group is carefully planned and worked out.
9. Durability	The groups are relatively durable.	Groups may be temporary or permanent.
10. Effect on perso-nality	The group has a long-lasting influence upon the perso-nality development of members. Important for the child in his social develop-ment (Socialisation).	The impact of the group on the personality of the members is rather limited.
11. Nature of group control	Primary groups control the behaviour of the members to a great extent. Informal means of social control are enough to regulate the relations.	Secondary groups have limited control over the behaviour of the members Informal means are not enough and hence formal means of social control are resorted to for maintaining the group control.
12. "We" feeling	Each person is a primary group has "We feeling" of belonging to one unit.	No strong "We" feeling.

In-groups and Out-groups

Summer in his book "Folkways" has introduced a two-fold classification—"In-groups" and "Out-groups". The group to which an individual belongs or feels that he belongs is an "in-group" and the rest of the groups are "out-groups". The classification is based on differences such as family, caste, religion or culture. The In-group is referred to as "we". The out-group is indicated as "they" There is every chance of conflicts between such groups, e.g. class, caste conflicts. One of the aims of the Indian Republic is to build a classess and casteless society.

Group Structure

In primary group, the group structure is informal unlike in the secondary group where the group structure is formal and is regulated by formal rules. In the secondary group, statuses and roles, powers and rights of members are clearly defined. In the primary group, members are not particular about their rights and powers. The primary group is not well "organised" in the modern sense.

The primary group has a well defined boundary. Being small in number, the members move within the specified boundary. The secondary group with a large population, has larger spatial structure.

Intergroup Relationship

An individual may belong to many groups without actually meeting any of their other members. In hospitals, the nursing staff forms one group of whom only a few ever meet face to face at any one time. The nursing staff forms a separate group from the medical staff or the domestic staff or the maintenance staff, who have their own groups. The hospital staff as a whole, however, also forms a group with interests and activities concerning all. Nurses may at the same time, belong to a professional organisation such as Trained Nurses Association of India (TNAI) or Student Nurses Association (SNA). They may be also members of a political party or members of their religious sect. These larger groups are the secondary groups. In each group different demands may be made upon the nurse; sometimes these are conflicting and create anxiety until the difficulties are resolved.

Group Cycle

During their existence, the groups go through phases of development similar to growth and development stages of human beings. These are early difficulties of group formation and establishment of group norms which resemble childhood and adolescent troubles.

Groups have a period of adult maturity and finally develop the sluggishness of old age and the degenerative process of senility. This description refers to the functioning of the group as a whole and not to any individual members. Group standards are formed by the interaction. Once standards are made, the individual members are affected by them.

Group Behaviour

Group behaviour is also known as social behaviour.

Within a group, decisions about group actions or about group acceptance or rejection of particular points of view are routinely undertaken. There can be vigorous arguement and violent disagreement within the group without damage to "We feeling". The ultimate purpose is a change for the better. But when a group is criticized or attacked by an outsider it reacts as a whole by closing its ranks and protecting itself. For example, there may be violent disagreement between members of a political party. But the party will present a united front to outsiders. No change of views is likely to occur as a result of outside pressure on a group; on the contrary, the opinions harden and the group becomes rigid in its ideas, when it is attacked.

Groups are more efficient in solving problems than are the individual members. Small groups have been experimentally engaged in solving puzzles. It is seen that, while within a given time no single individual could solve the problems, groups were successful in providing the correct answer. This can happen only when every member concentrated on the problem. Committees become more competent than individuals in solving complex problems of the hospital when everybody is motivated with the same aim.

In discussion groups or committees, the contribution of each member is important. Often the silent members assess all the contributions made by the more vocal members. During the discussion, he may show approval or disapproval, look interested or bored. When at the end, the silent member speaks, his contribution may be of great importance.

When a decision has been made by a whole group, the members feel much more bound by the decision than it had been imposed on the group by one person. In making any attempts to help young mothers to change their way of feeding their infants, discussion groups are more effective than advice by the health visitor. Decisions about nursing procedures are more likely to be carried out if they are made by the ward sisters themselves.

Group Morale in Hospitals

In hospitals, when the morale is good, there will be outspoken and frank criticism from within, while all the members have the same aim of improving the existing practices. When an outsider criticises, all the staff are united in their defence. Group rules are generally accepted and implemented easily. But when a group's morale is low, discussion is generally avoided. People feel uneasy with each other. They cannot safely reveal their feelings and consequently hide them and avoid all controversies. This results in the group's inability to deal with its business. The most important points in the agenda are not discussed at all or dwelt with briefly while time is spent on unimportant issues.

Much of the knowledge about groups is derived from the therapeutic groups with mentally ill patients or from study of industrial relations. Studies of morale have established that the similar forces are present in hospital and industry. Unlike in industry, conflicts among hospital staff are not because of differences in policy or value systems. The conflict arises from the way staff evaluates their own and other people's contributions.

The ward sisters may feel that the doctors do not pay enough attention to their advice; student nurses may feel that the ward sisters do not recognise their contribution to patient care. While the ward sister may feel that the nursing superintendent does not listen to her problems, junior nurses may feel the same way about the ward sister and patients may feel that nobody listens to them.

This process of "information blockage" leads to high levels of anxiety among nurses which can be remedied when the problem is faced by the entire staff. Adherence to routine reduces the need for decision-making and relieves the individual nurse of this responsibility. The hierarchical structure among nursing staff delegates responsibility and removes it from any one person.

QUESTIONS

1. Define social groups. Explain the nature and characteristics of primary social group and its importance in society.
2. Describe the functions of primary and secondary groups.
3. What are the features of primary groups?
4. What are the characteristics of secondary groups?
5. Give two examples of social groups.
6. Give two examples each of primary and secondary groups.
7. Compare and contrast primary groups and secondary groups.
8. In modern society, secondary groups are as important as primary groups. Explain how?
9. What are "In groups" and what are their characteristics?

24 Social Changes and Social Control

Change is the law of life. Every society must change with passage of time. Social change is the change in society. Society is a web of social relationships. Hence, social change is a change in social relationships. Social relationships are understood in terms of social processes and social interactions and social organisation. The term "social change" is used to describe variations in social interactions, social processes and social organisation. It includes alterations in the structure and functions of the society. In the words of ME Jones, "social change is a term used to describe variations or modifications of any aspect of social process, social pattern, social interactions or social organisation". Thus, social change is a change in the social organisation.

Nature of Social Change

1. Social change is a universal phenomenon. No society remains completely static.
2. Social change is community change. It is not a change in the life of an individual but it is a change that occurs in the life of the entire community.
3. Speed of social change is not uniform in every society. In most societies, it occurs so slowly that it is often not noticed. Social changes in urban areas are faster than in rural areas. The speed of social change in each age or period is not the same in the same society.
4. Social change occurs either in the natural course or as a result of planned action. Our needs keep on changing. For changing needs social change is a necessity.

5. Definite prediction of social change is not possible. It cannot be predicted what shall be ideas, attitudes, norms and values in future.
6. Social changes may create chain reactions. Change in one aspect of life may lead to a series of changes in other aspects. For example, change in rights, privileges and status of women has resulted in a series of changes in home and family relationships.
7. Social change may be planned or unplanned. Plans, programmes and projects may be launched by man in order to determine and control the rate and direction of social change. Unplanned change refers to change resulting from natural calamitics like famines, floods, earthquakes, etc.
8. Social changes are chiefly those of modification or of replacement. It may be modification of physical goods or social relationships. Our ideas about women's rights and coeducation stand modified today.

Change also takes the form of replacement. Bullock carts have been replaced by automobiles. Similarly, old ideas have been replaced by new ideas. The germ theory has replaced the older theories about cause of diseases. Democracy has replaced aristocracy.

Factors Affecting Social Changes

1. *Geographical factor* changes in the geographical environment create changes in social life. Floods, earthquakes, drought, volcano eruptions, etc. bring about important changes to society. Continuous floods may give rise to new townships. The earthquake at Koyna dam site forced to build a new township. The great volcanic eruption of Yokohama in 1923 was responsible for a new kind of architecture in Japan.
2. *Biological factor:* Intercaste marriages and interreligious marriages produce a new type of human growth with different mental and physical outlook. Demographic factor means size and composition of population. A small society may not have a place in history but a large society leaves historical evidence of its culture.

3. *Technological factor:* Scientific discoveries inventions and new machinery bring about revolutionary changes in society. For example, the introduction of steam, electric and petrol driven machines for production, transport and communication have drastically changed our material environment influencing social changes.
4. *Economic factors:* Man has to struggle for his living. There are basic norms that govern the economic relations among people. The mode of production determines the general character of social, political and economic aspects of life. According to Karl Marx, a day will come when there will be no class or caste ridden society.
5. *Culture factor:* There is an intimate relationship between our beliefs and institutions, values and social relationships. Thus, the social and cultural aspects are so closely interwoven that all cultural changes lead to social changes.

A static society is more harmful than of any advantage to its members. Though social change is a universal phenomenon, in no society changes are accepted without opposition or resistance.

Social Control

Social control is defined as any influence which the society exerts upon its members for the purpose of providing security to the group as a whole. It is the way in which members of the society are made to conform to the social norms (rules of conduct). Types of social control are: (a) Informal, (b) Formal:

Informal (Indirect) Means of Social Control

1. *Belief:* It is the conviction that a particular thing is true such as belief in the existence of an unseen power, belief in the theory of rebirth, belief in the existence of heaven and hell. Beliefs have powerful influences on human actions.
2. *Social suggesions:* It is the indirect communication of ideas, and feelings. We celebrate Gandhi Jayanthi and build monuments for great men. We place their life and ideals before the people for them to follow. Advertisements are very, powerful tools of imparting social suggestions to do or not to do certain things.

3. *Ideologies:* Ideology is a social theory of life which interprets social realities from the points of new of ideals. Leninism has influenced the social life of the Russians. Gandhism has influenced the social life in India. Ideologies stimulate action and provide a set of values for social action. They make life meaningful.
4. *Folkways:* These are the recognised modes of behaviour which arise automatically within a group. They are the behaviour patterns of everyday life. They are foundation of group culture. They are socially approved and become a habit and followed unconsciously. Brahmins do not eat meat, Muslims do not eat pork, Jains do not eat curd, Sikhs do not smoke. All these and other folkways (ways of the folk) are social in nature and are of unplanned origin. They save our time and energy and add some regularity and definiteness to our behaviour.
5. *Mores pronounced "movaes" (singular 'mos'):* Mores are those folkways, which are considered by the group to be indispensable for the welfare of the group. They relate more to the fundamental needs of the society than folkways. They express the group sense of what is right and conductive to social welfare. For example, prohibition, endogamy, monogamy, anti-slavery "when the folkways have added to the conceptions of group welfare, standards of right and wrong, they are converted into mores"-MacIver. Mores are included in the normative system of the group and in the laws of the state. For example, patriotism, devotion and love for parents, concern for one's own children, faithfulness of husband and wife to each other.
6. *Customs:* Customs are long established habits and usages of the people. They are those mores and folkways existed for a very long time and passed on from generation to generations. They arise spontaneously and gradually and regulate social life to a great extent. For example, caste, endogamy, child marriage, taboo on widow remarriage, dowry system and untouchability are some of the customs of the Hindu society. Girls after marriage join the husbands' family and boys look after old parents.
7. *Habits:* Habits are developed by individuals by repeating certain action until they are done without conscious effort. Good habits

like hygiene, eating, sleeping, etc. should be taught to children. Bad habits like smoking, drinking or drug abuse should be avoided.

8. *Religion:* Religion is an attitude towards super human powers. It is a powerful agency in society and influences human behaviour. It makes children obey their parents, makes people benevolent, charitable and truthful.
9. *Art and Literature:* The martial music of military band arouses feelings of determination and strength, Ramayana and Mahabhartha are works of high social value. Dickens changed the education system of England by his novels "David Copperfield" and "Oliver Twist".
10. *Humour and Satire:* Humour assumes various forms depending on the situation and purpose. Satire employs scorn as indirect criticism of harmful behaviour of people and causes the erring people to give up their vicious and harmful ways.
11. *Public opinion:* For fear of pubic opinion and criticism people avoid immoral and antisocial activities. The influence of public opinion as a means of social control is greater in simple societies. In a village, all the people are known to each other personally, so it is difficult for a villager to act contrary to the public opinion of the village. Public opinion greatly influences all our activities. Every individual wants to win public praise (recognition) and avoid public ridicule or criticism.

Differences between Folkways and Mores

a. Folkways are the general ways of behaviour (for example wearing different dresses for different occasions, walking on the left side of the road, eating three meals a day) while mores are obligatory ways of behaviour.
b. Values of right and wrong are not well defined in folkways unlike in mores.
c. When folkways are not followed mild reproof (disapproval) is expressed by society but when mores are broken, severe punishment follows.
d. Mores are much more powerful agencies of social control than are the folkways.

e. Folkways may be changed according to individual taste. For example, one may greet another by folded hands or handshake. There is generally no such choice in mores.

Formal Means of Social Control

1. *Law*: Informal means of social control are not sufficient to control large modern societies and laws are made to define the expected standards of behaviour and punishments to be imposed on those who violate the rules and regulations.
2. *Education:* Education is a process of socialization. It prepares the child for social living.
3. *Coersion (compulsion):* Physical coersion is the lowest form of social control. Non-violent coersion consists of strike, boycot and non-cooperation.

QUESTIONS

1. Explain the process of socialisation.
2. Define social change. Explain its characteristics.
3. Describe the factors that resist social change.
4. Define social change. Discuss briefly the various factors of social change with examples.
5. What are the consequences of social change?
6. Describe the factors for social change.
7. Describe how education brings about social change.
8. What are the agencies of social control? Explain each one of them.
9. What is social control? Explain what are formal and informal means of social control.
10. Explain how customs and laws act as agencies of social control.
11. Examine the characteristics and importance of folkways.
12. Explain the characteristics and importance of mores.
13. Distinguish between laws, folkways and mores.
14. Describe the importance of social norms.

25 Social Stratification: Rural and Urban Society

No two individuals are exactly alike. Diversity and inequality are inherent in society. Hence, human society is everywhere stratified.

Stratification is the process by which individuals and groups are ranked in a more or less enduring hierarchy of status. According to RW Mury, social stratification is horizontal division of society into higher and lower social units.

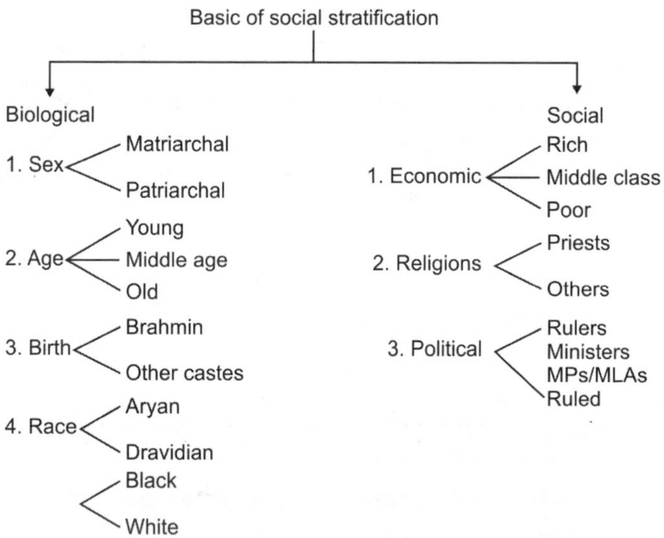

Social Stratification in India: The Caste System

The caste system, as a form of social stratification is peculiar to India. The English word caste is derived from Portuguese (also Spanish) word "casta" meaning lineage or race.

Caste is a hereditary type of social group. The Hindu social order is based on the caste system. The group or caste has a common name and a traditional occupation. The membership is by birth. The members have many castes within their own groups (sub-castes) or else be treated as outcastes. The rules about food and drink are very strict. There is the idea of pollution by touch, e.g. wells are said to be polluted when untouchables use them.

Brahmins are the highest class, followed by Khatriyas, Vyshays and Sudras (Chaturvarna) Untouchables with no caste are even lower in social status. Mahatma Gandhi named them Harijans and worked for the removal of untouchability. Still they are made to live separately outside the village. The lowest and the most depressed are the scheduled castes. To help them move up the social ladder, they are given opportunities and reservations in education and employment. There is an "Untouchability Offence Act" to prevent any ill treatment to the untouchables.

Merits of the Caste System

1. *Definite social environment:* It provides a definite social environment to its members. Culture of each caste is different from the other.
2. *Spirit of cooperation:* There is a sense of "we feeling" among the members of each caste. Because of "we feeling" cooperation is automatically developed.
3. *It defines economic persuit:* The caste system determines the occupation of its members. The young ones are given training by the parents and other elder members of their caste.
4. *Racial purity:* Caste system maintains racial purity by prohibiting intercaste marriages. Culture of each caste remains pure.
5. *Provides for various functions:* It provides for various functions necessary to social life—functions ranging from education to scavenging. It provides a much better division of labour than the European class system.
6. *Cultural diffusion:* It helps in cultural diffusion within the group. The customs, beliefs, skills, behaviour and trade secrets are passed on from generation to generation. Culture is thus carried from one age to another.

7. *Separation of social from political life:* Caste system distinctively separates social life from political influence. Many invaders of the country, for example, the Muslims and Western people tried to convert native Hindus to their religion but caste system prevented mass conversions.

Demerits of Caste System

1. *No scope for social mobility:* The caste system does not encourage mobility of labour. It provides limited opportunity to change their social status.
2. *Untouchability:* Caste hierachy leads to the feeling of superiority and untouchability. Persons of higher castes consider the Sudras as subhuman and think that very touch of sudra will pollute them. Social barriers were erected and the people of lower castes were not given opportunities for physical and mental development. Many lower caste people got themselves converted to Islam, Christianity and Budhism and Budhism due to the brutalities of the upper castes.
3. *Social disunity:* Caste system with hundreds of castes and subcastes has developed hatred and enemity to other castes. The system encouraged antisocial conducts. Crimes committed by higher castes were not punished.
4. *Wrong men for jobs:* In the caste system, some particular occupations were alloted to a particular caste without looking into its ability to perform. Members of one caste were forbidden to take an occupation alloted to another caste. This has placed a wrong man in a wrong occupation which retarded economic progress.
5. *Hindrance to national unity:* A modern nation can become strong only on the principles of liberty, equality and fraternity. Caste system is opposite to these ideas. It has proved to be a great stumbling block to national integration. India could not develop a strong feeling of nationality.
6. *Status:* The status of persons were graded in the hierarchy. From the very birth, some were made inferior and others superior. Individual freedom was denied to the down trodden and justice was denied to them. Inequality was made a social system.

7. *Moral degradation:* The system encouraged antisocial conduct because there were separate laws for the previledged. People from higher castes were not punished. The system encouraged untouchability and sati and other evils.
8. *Undemocratic:* The caste system is undemocratic as it denies equal rights to all.

Disintegration of Caste System in India
Future of Caste System in India

Buddhism, Jainism, Islam, Christianity and Sikhism condemned the rigidity of Hindu caste system but could not alter it.

1. *Reformist movements:* The spread of Western education is an important factor to reduce the influence of the caste system in India. Several reform movements like Arya Samaj, Brahma Samaj, Veerashaivism, Bhakti movement and Ramakrishna Mission tried to denounce the caste declaring that it had no religious sanction. Mahatma Gandhi struggled hard to eradicate the evil of untouchability in India and for promoting communal harmony.
2. *Legislation during British period:* The British brought with them a casteless culture and promoted individual liberty. The British government passed various laws like Widow Remarriage Act and Caste Disabilities Removal Act which weakened the caste system. By establishing British Courts and administering uniform criminal law, they removed from the caste panchayats many matters that used be dwelt by them. The lower castes were forbidden from public places like temples, public wells and hotels and suffered from many social disabilities.
3. *Industrialisation:* Industrial revolution has also been a factor responsible for transforming the Hindu social structure. It provided uniform work styles and division of labour. Migration of more people from rural to industrial cities caused a break in the traditional caste ideas. Ascribed status of castes occupations changed to achieve status by performance of work. Family and kinship groups which were once the units of production were affected by the new industrial system. Industrialisation caused

urbanisation in which people of all caste groups mingled with new ideas of commercialism and entertainment.

4. *Attack by Indian constitution:* Indian constitution inaugurated on 26th January 1950 proclaimed India as a Sovereign Democratic Republic with the main aim of creating a casteless and classless society. In guaranteeing the right of equality. Sec 15 of the constitution reads:
5. i. The state shall not discriminate any citizen on grounds only of religion, race, caste, sex, place of birth or any of them.
   ii. No citizen shall, on grounds only of religion, race, caste, sex, place of birth or any of them, be subject to any disability, liability, restriction or condition with regard to:
      a. Access to shops, public restaurants, hotels and places of public entertainment or
      b. The use of wells, tanks, bathing ghats, roads and places of public entertainment maintained wholly or partly out of state funds or dedicated to the use of general public.

Future of Caste System in India

Though the influence of caste system is steadily decreasing, it is still very powerful as there is very little change in the attitude and mentality of people. There have been anti Brahminical movements in Maharashtra, Tamil Nadu, Karnataka and many other states. The rise of Mahars and Marathas as political groups in Maharashtra, Kammas and Reddys in Andhra Pradesh, DK and DMK movements in Tamil Nadu, Lingayats and Vokkaligas in Karnataka are for achievement of power and pre-eminence.

There has been a tendency towards formation of caste associations particularly among lower caste groups. The elections in India are contested very much on the basis of castes. Political parties sponsor only candidates whose caste is numerous in that area.

The voters are asked to vote for their caste candidates and thus casteism is maintained by the elected leaders after elections are over. Casteism still persists in government services and in legislatures.

QUESTIONS

1. Define social stratification and show its peculiar nature in India.
2. What is social stratification?
3. Define caste. State any one function of "Caste Panchayats"?
4. Explain any four traditional characteristics of caste.
5. Define class and caste. Discuss the caste system in India.
6. Explain the adverse effects of caste. What are its consequences on health.
7. Describe the causes that have contributed to the changes of the caste system in modern India.
8. Explain the new roles of caste system in independent India.
9. Briefly describe social stratification. What are the differences between social stratification and social classification?
10. Discuss the various social problems confronting the Indian villages.
11. Explain the rural development programmes initiated by the government during the recent years.
12. Briefly examine the changes that are taking place in the Indian villages during the recent years.
13. Explain the three rural development programmes undertaken by the government during recent years.
14. What are health problems of Indian village community?
15. What are the health aspects of social problems?

26 Social Problems

UNMARRIED MOTHERS

Due to the selfishness of men, girls are lured into sexual activity before marriage and they become pregnant causing problems to themselves, their parents and the society at large. This problem was less in olden days when premarital sex was considered a sin and age of marriage was much lower. Today men and women work together in offices and factories and have lot of chances to meet privately. Late marriage on the part of women and men also leads to premarital relationships. Sometimes ignorance about sex may also result in unmarried mothers.

Many societies abroad take a lineant view of premarital and extramarital sexual relationships but not so in India. But the unwed mothers need sympathy and help from the society and state. Instead of condemning them, the society must find out the causes of their problem and solve them. In advanced countries, unwed mothers are given free food, accommodation and other benefits, so that they and their infants will not suffer from malnutrition and diseases.

The unwed mothers should be given the choice to retain the child. Otherwise social organizations should look after the child and its legal adoption. Becoming an unwed mother should not be serious handicap in the future life of such unfortunate individuals.

DOWRY SYSTEM

Dowry refers to money, goods, gifts or estate that the wife brings to her husband in marriage. The Dowry Prohibition Act 1961, defines it as "any property or valuable security which might be given or agreed to be given either directly or indirectly by one party in marriage to the other party in marriage either by themselves or through parents or through any other person which may be presented either before or at the time of marriage or even after that."

Dowry is a major problem of marriage in India in most communities. With increasing importance of money, the amount of dowry is on the increase inspite of spread of education and enlightenment.

Causes of Dowry

1. Difficulty to find a suitable groom
2. Child marriage
3. Dowry as a prestige symbol
4. Not so very good looking girls
5. Absolute necessity of marriage as per Hindu scriptures
6. For stability of marriage
7. The custom of Kanyadan
8. Desire to marry from rich families
9. Materialistic outlook in life
10. Accepting dowry in son's marriage to spend in daughter's marriage as dowry.

Evils of Dowry System

1. Parents take heavy loans to marry off their daughters
2. Suicide by young girls not to become a financial burden to their parents
3. Girls remain unmarried
4. Female infanticides
5. Child marriages
6. Unmatched and incompatible marriages
7. Constant quarrels and dowry deaths.
8. Low status of women. A girl child is considered as a burden and curse. She is not educated properly. She is looked down upon in her husband's family, if she does not bring a fat dowry.

Dowry Prohibition Act 1961

Attempts have been made to eradicate the evil dowry system. Gandhiji was much against dowry and he educated youth to be self-dependent and take pledge not to accept dowry. Dowry Prohibition Act 1961 was passed by Central Government in 1961. Gifts given at the time of marriage are not included in dowry. This is a serious drawback. The complaint is to be made within one year of paying the dowry. The crime is not cognizable. Punishment is imprisonment of minimum six months which may extent to two years and a fine upto ₹ 10,000/- (Rupees ten thousands only).

Remedial Measures: Some Suggestions

1. Encourage intercaste marriages
2. Educate girls and make them economically independent
3. Equal share to girls in father's property
4. Encourage boys to stand on their own feet and then marry
5. Young people should take pledge against dowry
6. More effective legislation.

PROSTITUTION

This is another social problem related to women. It is an ancient social evil and is more common in Urban areas.

The causes for becoming a prostitute may be similar to those causing boys to become delinquent. The causes may be (1) Death of parents, lack of education, lack of occupation and poverty (2) She wants money to dress well or to gain financial help to family (3) Eloping with false lover and ultimately take to prostitution (4) Because of shame when she becomes pregnant without being married (5) A drug addict may want money through prostitution for purchasing the drugs (6) Kidnapping or someone in the trade promising a job in the city. Soon the unfortunate girls are imprisoned in a brothel along with other girls and forced to give sexual pleasure for money. Once a person enters it, she may never come out. There is a pimp who exploits her and the "Madam" who keeps the house and takes away the major part of the earnings. Prostitution is a business enterprise.

Evil Effects

1. *The spread of venereal diseases and AIDS* is a most serious menace.
2. *Disturbance of family relationship:* Prostitution causes domestic disharmony due to venereal diseases and marital unfaithfulness.
3. *Personal demoralization:* Practically every study of prostitutes shows a progressive deterioration of ideals. They become hard hearted, incapable of loving anyone. They start suspecting everyone and finally loose their faith in mankind.
4. Prostitution as a commercial proposition requires a number of men for one woman. It is an act of perversity.

The government of India has passed the Suppression of Immoral Traffic Act in women and girls in 1956 to control prostitution. The Act was amended and retitled as "Immoral Traffic (Prevention) Act in 1986. Raids are being made on brothels and girls taken to jail, but it is not difficult for the brothel keeper to pay and get back these girls. Rehabilitation programes are needed to help the girls and limit the problem. Only when poverty is alleviated, and women who had gone astray are treated with sympathy and given good education, can we eradicate this evil. Further, the state should provide them with alternate jobs to live with honour and dignity in the society.

DRUG ADDICTION

The word "drug" is defined as any substance that when taken by a living organism may modify one or more of its functions (WHO) when a drug can alter consciousness, it is called a psychoactive drug. A psychoactive drug acts directly upon the brain. It can change our ability to focus attention, remember things, use judgement, have a sense of time, control our actions and emotions. Drugs may be: (1) Stimulants (2) Depressants or, (3) Hallucinogens.

1. *A stimulant or "upper"* alters consciousness because it makes us feel good and more alert, e.g. caffeine, nicotine, cocaine and ametamines.
2. *A depressant or "downer"* is just the reverse of stimulant. It alters the consciousness by depressing the central nervous system

and make people more relaxed and less tense. Examples are alcohol, barbiturates and marijuana (Pot or grass).

3. *Hallucinogens* are drugs which cause a person to have hallucinations or visions, e.g. LSD (Lysergic acid dimethylamine) hashish, ganja, bhang. Although some have pleasurable dreams when using LSD, majority has very bad experiences with destructive behaviour and loss of orientation.

Drug addiction is defined as a state of periodic or chronic intoxication detrimental to the individual and society produced by the repeated intake of habit forming drugs.

To call a person a drug addict, the following criteria must be satisfied:

1. *Psychologic dependence:* There is an overpowering desire (compulsion) to take the drug and obtain it by any means.
2. *Physical dependence:* When the drug in withdrawn, the patient shows "withdrawal symptoms" such as irrational or violent behaviour, nausea, diarrhoea, watering of the eye and nose.
3. *Development of tolerance:* There is a tendency to increase the dose.

Simultaneously with medical treatment, changes in environment (home, school, college, social circle) are important. The patient must effect a complete break with his group to avoid the sure relapse.

Preventive measures include education of target group through TV, radio, postures and leaflets to create awareness of the problem. The government have promulgated an act called the "Narcotic Drugs and Psychotropic substances Act which came into force in 1985 to deal with drug addiction.

ALCOHOLISM

Alcoholism like drug addiction affects not only the health and welfare of the individual, but of the family and society at large.

Alcoholism is characterised by four factors:

1. Excessive intake of alcoholic beverages
2. Individual's increasing worry over his drinking.

3. Loss of the drinker's control over his drinking.
4. Disturbances in his social life.

Consequences of alcohol abuse: Excessive consumption of alcohol harm the human body in different ways. By its action on the brain, it blocks functions like sensation, perception and reasoning; by its action on the stomach, it causes gastritis, by its action on the liver, it causes cirrhosis of the liver and its action on the heart may produce hypertension and heart failure.

Alcohol abuses cause many evils such as crime, murder, prostitution, neglect of families, malnutrition, disease, unemployment, indebtedness, child delinquency, road accidents, loss of friends and selfesteem.

Over the past fifty years, alcohol consumption has increased both in quantity and frequency. The age at which people start drinking has also declined. The population at great risk are those undergoing rapid socioeconomic and cultural changes. They view alcohol as a symbol of prestige and social status. Drinking by adults serves as a role model for the young.

Treatment

Deadiction cannot take place unless the individual willingly come forward and attend the deadiction programme. Unfortunately most alcoholics are not motivated to undergo treatment. While many deny that their alcohol consumption is abnormal, others openly defend their habits.

Identification of the risk factor is essential for prevention. As drinking patterns vary considerably, the prevention of alcoholism is not easy. Long-term treatment is not only a medical problem and needs the cooperation of psychologists and sociologists as well. There is also the problem of high relapse rate with all treatment methods.

A widespread public education and discussion and investigation of public attitudes may result in considerable improvement. This should be combined with social welfare and health services.

DELINQUENCY

Juvenile delinquency is antisocial behaviour committed by young people who is under an age specified by the law of the land. According to juvenile justice Act of 1986, the prescribed age is 18 years for both boys and girls. Juvenile delinquents are underaged or non-adult criminals who engage in offences that constitute crimes if committed by adults. Antisocial practices of this type are very dangerous to the welfare of the society.

Causes for antisocial behaviour (delinquency) are:

a. Environmental factors
b. Personality factors.

Environmental Factors

1. Low economic income
2. Living in a transitional area
3. Family breakdown.

Delinquency is the highest in areas which are in a process of transition or migration. When a family disintegrates, child is deprived of affection, feelings of security and social opportunities. If such a child comes in contact with a delinquent gang that can satisfy some of his needs, the child may follow that gang and become delinquent. Among mothers, it has been found that those who had been divorced or separated enhibited more anger and non-conformity.

Personality Factors

Delinquents find difficulty in correctly interpreting and evaluating both their behaviour and the behaviour of others. They are morally blind. Once a person has comitted a crime, the chances of committing another crime are very high. Low educational background and poverty are the most important causes of delinquency. If is more an urban than a rural phenomenon. Metropolitan cities produce more delinquents than small cities and towns. Delinquency rates are higher among boys than girls and is highest during early adolescence (12–16 age group).

Causes of juvenile delinquency in India:

1. Poverty and child abuse
2. Breakdown of joint family
3. Breakdown of religious influences and moral values
4. Illiteracy and lack of education.
5. Industrialisation and urbanisation, together with large scale migration to cities.
6. Absence of proper facilities for marriage and family counselling, so as to have responsible and mature parent-hood.
7. Political problems
8. Social changes.

Serious forms of juvenile delinquency in India:

1. Damaging and stealing property
2. Murder, assault and suicide
3. Sexual offences like rape and sodomy
4. Escape from custody
5. Ticketless travel in trains
6. Gambling.

Remedial Measures

1. A proper assessment of the problem as per scientific principles of sociology.
2. Improvement in economic conditions of the masses.
3. Provision of better education facilities
4. Training for parents in parental responsibility
5. Encouraging religion and morality
6. Facilities for proper treatment and reformation of juvenile delinquents, with the provision of juvenile courts, juvenile police and reformation centres.

Criminologists believe that an adult who is habitual criminal cannot be rehabilited. Prevention must start early if it is to be effective. Community planning (social institutions, social workers, etc.) and judicial action should start early as preventive measures.

THE HANDICAPPED

A handicapped child is one who deviates from normal child physically, mentally and psychologically:

1. *Physically handicapped:*
   a. Blind, deaf, dumb or cleft palate
   b. Crippled by cerebral palsy, polio-affected
   c. Burns-affected
   d. Children with heart diseases.
2. *Mentally handicapped:*
   a. Feeble minded
   b. Mentally retarded.
3. *Psychologically handicapped:*
   a. Neglected orphans, deprived and abandoned
   b. Children deprived of parents affection
   c. Maladjusted, delinquent with behaviour problems.

Education of Handicapped Children

The goal is to help the handicapped child and his family, so that the child may lead a normal life and self-supporting and useful member of the society Helen Keller and Stephen Hawkin are outstanding examples of people with many handicaps but with outstanding contributions to society. Health and social authorities, welfare and educational agencies all need to work together to reach the goal of special education.

Visually challenged children must be referred early to a special school and taught through Braille system. Most schools for the blind give training (rehabilitation) in walking independently with the specially marked cane. They also provide training in weaving, basket making, cane knitting and other skills.

Deaf children also can be trained in special schools; some of them can be helped with hearing aids. Many do well in certain occupations and become useful citizens; same is true of the mentally challenged. However, some of them may need a sheltered environment.

Nurses who are in charge of handicapped children should behave in such a way that the children do not feel that they are disabled and develop an inferiority complex. They should be made to feel that with a little effort they can also become useful citizens and not a burden on society. They are differently abled and not disabled.

Rehabilitation Centres

These centres provide specialized facilities for physically handicapped children as follows:

1. Physical therapy, special exercises and electrical therapy to strengthen muscles.
2. Fitting of artificial limps or calipers.
3. Occupational therapy to teach painting, music, book binding and weaving.
4. Speech therapy for needy children.

CRIMES AGAINST WOMEN IN INDIA

Crimes against women include violence against women, rape, molestation, dowry harassment, wife-battering, kidnapping female children to be sold into brothel homes, forced marriage, forcible religious conversion, immoral traffic in women, killing female children in the foetus stage, harassment of women at the workplace including eve teasing, negligence of women's health and education. These crimes have doubled during the last ten years. Majority of women in India are not after equality with men but they want a respectable and meaningful position for them in the society. But no radical change in the status of women of India is likely because of:

1. Continued male supremacy
2. Regional, caste, and communal differences
3. Women exploiting women
4. Lack of powerful organizations and movements of women
5. No protection for the interests of lower caste and class women
6. Indifferent attitude of the government and political leaders.

QUESTIONS

1. Discuss the various social problems and their causes.
2. List the various social problems of urban community.

3. Write short notes on:
   a. Drug addiction and alcoholism.
   b. Health hazards of alcoholism.
   c. Handicapped
   d. Unmarried mothers
   e. Prostitution
   f. Dowry
4. What is delinquency? Explain its causes.

27 Social Agencies and Remedial Measures

Society controls social behaviour and social relationships. This is carried out through agencies like family, religion and law.

Family

Family is a living social system. Although it is a basic unit of society, it is a sub system as it is regarded as one of the parts of the society which is a larger social system. Family is primary group of individuals who are interdependent. Therefore, the choice and actions of one family member often influence all other family members. For example, when one member of the family is ill, the entire family is affected.

Religion as a Social Institution

Man is a religious or spiritual being. Religion provides an opportunity for the individual for attaining spiritual experiences of prayer, meditation and worship. It provides peace of mind, emotional support, faith, hope, optimism and courage. It explains individual suffering and helps to integrate the personality. It conserves moral, spiritual and social values and promotes welfare activities like mutual help, sympathy and cooperation.

Society Welfare services have always been an integral part of the social cultural tradition of India. Several social welfare services are intended to cater to the weaker sections of the population. These include women, children, handicapped, aged, scheduled castes and tribes. The department of social welfare was created in 1964 under Central Government to look after general social welfare. It plans and coordinates the welfare services run by the

Government of India, State Governments and National Voluntary agencies. Activities include welfare, training, health care, provision of women's hostels, as well as legal aid and support to women being exploited by families and employers.

A few of the principal agencies for women are:

1. All India Women's Conference
2. National Association of Rural Women
3. National Council for Women
4. Centre of Science for Villages
5. Indian Social Institute, Department of Women's Development
6. Eastern India Women's Association
7. Family Planning Association of India
8. Kasturaba Gandhi Trust
9. Kamala Nehru Memorial Trust
10. Indira Gandhi Trust.

Child Welfare

Children contribute 40% of India's population Article 25 of Indian constitution lays down that no child below the age of 14 shall be employed to work in any factory or mine of hazardous nature. India adopted its national policy on children in 1974. On October 2, 1975, the integrated child development services (ICDS) were introduced to implement the national policy on children. Right to free education for children upto 14 years of age has been made compulsory with effect from 1st April, 2010.

Welfare of the Old People

Once the aged commanded great respect due to the traditional norms and values of Indian society but due to disintegration of joint family system and the recent changes in family values, the generation gap has widened. The elderly people are neglected by their own children and they feel unwanted.

The problem of the aged can be mitigated by providing necessary welfare facilities to them by way of (i) Reasonable amount of old age pension, (ii) Free medical care, (iii) Housing facilities in the form of old age homes, (iv) Recreational facilities to relieve their loneliness and (v) The usual courtesies extended to them.

There are numerous voluntary organisation like Help Age India and Age Care India who are very active and helpful in the care of the aged.

Help Age India was established in 1978 on the pattern of Help the Aged Society of England. It is a voluntary organisation working nationwide for the cause and care of the elder people with its Head office in New Delhi with a network of 22 centres in major cities. Besides creating awareness among the young generation about the needs of the aged in the society, it also conducts sponsored events like painting competitions, debates, grandparents meet, etc. It collects funds and provide facilities including items for the Aged, geriatric wards, mobile medicare units, rehabilitation of the aged, blind, cataract operations, leprosy patients and physically handicapped.

Social security: Social security is defined as that security that the society furnishes though appropriate organisations against certain risks to which the members are exposed. The risks which social security covers in most countries are sickness, invalidity, maternity, old age and death. Social security also includes social insurance and social assistance.

Social security for industrial workers are contained in the following legislations:

1. Workmen's Compensation Act, 1923
2. Employees State Insurance Act, 1948
3. Central Maternity Benefit Act, 1961
4. The family Pension Scheme 1971.

Social Security for Civil Servants

Employees of the Central and State Governments have pension, gratuity, provident fund, group insurance and family pension schemes.

Social Security for the General Public

The risks of health, accident and fire are covered by insurance schemes. Life Insurance Corporation (LIC) of India has many schemes for general public. There are also public provident fund schemes.

QUESTIONS

1. Explain how family controls social behaviour and social relationship.
2. Explain the part played by religion as a social agency.
3. What are the three social agencies? Explain briefly each one of them.
4. Discuss the social welfare planning in India.
5. Give an account of the community development programme in India.

28 Community and Culture

DEFINITIONS OF COMMUNITY

"A social group with 'we feeling' and living in a given area"—Bagardus

"The smallest territorial group that can embrace all aspects of social life"—Kingsley Davis.

Meaning: A group of people inhabiting a given geographic area, sharing a common way of life, working together for certain ends, aware that they belong to the community as well as the larger society. People will have common interest and activities united together with common living pattern and organized social life.

Characteristics of Community

1. *Locality:* A community is a territorial group. It always occupies some geographic area. Locality is the physical area of a community. Even a wandering tribe or a nomad community, for example has a locality.
2. *Community sentiment:* Community sentiment means a feeling of belonging together. The members must be aware of their staying together and sharing common interests. The members develops a sense of "we feeling". It means a kind of identification with the group.

   Other characteristics of community
3. *Stability or relative permanence:* A community has not only locality and community sentiment, but has also stability. It is not a temporary group like a crowd or a mob. It is relatively stable. It includes a permanent group life in a definite place.
4. Community is established in a normal and natural way. They are not made or created by an act of will or by planned effort. Individuals become members of the community by birth.

5. *Size of the community:* The term community in a relative sense. There are bigger or wider communities which include small communities like villages, towns, cities or tribes.
6. *Regulation of relation:* Every community develops in course of time, a system of traditions, customs, morals and practices, a bundle of rules and regulations to regulate the relation of its members. In the rural community, informal means of social control is observed, e.g. folkways, customs, rituals, mores and beliefs.
7. *Dependency:* An individual in a community is physically dependent on community for satisfaction of physical needs. He is psychologically also dependent on the community because it saves him from the fear of solitude and boredom of isolation.

Society and Community—Differences

Society	Community
1. Society is a web of social relationships	1. Community consists of group of people living in a particular area with some degree of "we feeling"
2. A definite geographic area is not an essential aspect of society	2. Community always denotes a definite locality or geographic area
3. Society is abstract	3. Community is concrete
4. "Community sentiment" or a sense of "we feeling" may not be present in society	4. "Community sentiment" is an essential element of community. There can be no community without "we feeling"
5. Society involves both likeness and differences. Common interests as well as diverse interests are present in society	5. Likeness is more important than differences in community. There is common agreement of interests and objectives on the part of members
6. Society is wider. There can bemore than one community in a society	6. Community is smaller than society
7. The objectives and interests of society are more extensive and varied	7. The objectives and interests of a community are comparatively less extensive and varied

Types of Community

1. *Tribal community* consisting of mostly preliterate people living far away from the area of influence of civilization.
2. *Rural community* consisting of people living in villages, depending mainly on agriculture and allied occupations.
3. *Urban community* consisting of people living in towns and cities depending mainly on nonagricultural occupations.

CULTURE

The term culture is derived from the Latin word Cultura and Sanskrit word Samskar", which denotes social channel and intellectual excellence. Culture is a way of life.

Definitions

Edward B Taylor, the famous English anthropologist, has defined culture as "that complex whole which includes knowledge, belief, art, morals, law, custom and any other capabilities and habits acquired by man as a member of society (Primitive culture 1871).

B Malinowski has defined culture as the cumulative creation of man. He also regards culture as the handiwork of man and the medium through which he achieves his ends.

Graham Wallas, an English sociologist has defined culture as an accumulation of thoughts, values and objects. It is the social heritage acquired by us from preceding generations through learning, as distinguished from biological heritage which is passed on to us automatically through genes.

Characteristics of Culture

1. *Culture is social:* Culture is social and not an individual heritage of man. It does not exist in isolation. It is a product of society and shared by all the members of the society. No man can acquire culture without association with other human beings.
2. *Culture is learnt:* Culture is not inherited biologically, but learnt socially by man. It is not an inborn tendency.

There is no cultural instinct as such. Culture is often called learnt ways of behavior.

3. *Culture is shared:* Culture is not something that an individual can possess. For example, customs, traditions, beliefs, ideas, values and morals are shared by people of a group or society.
4. *Culture is transmissive:* Culture is transmitted vertically or horizontally and thus is communication. Vertical transmission is from generation to generation. Horizontal transmission is from one group to another group within the same period. Language is the chief vehicle of culture.
5. *Culture is continuous and cumulative:* Culture exists as a continuous process. It is the social heritage of man. It is linked with the past. The past endures because it lives in culture. In its historical growth, it tends to become cumulative. Culture is a "growing whole" which includes in itself, the achievements of the past and the present and makes provision for future achievements of mankind.
6. *Culture is consistent and integrated:* Culture is an integrated system. It preserves an order and system. At the same time, different parts of culture are interconnected. For example, the value system of society is closely connected with its other aspects like mortality, religion, customs, traditions and beliefs.
7. *Culture is dynamic and adaptive:* Though culture is relatively stable, it is not altogether static. It is subject to slow but constant changes. Culture is also responsive to changing condition of the physical world. It is adaptive. It also intervenes in the natural environment and helps man in his process of adjustment.
8. *Culture is gratifying:* Culture provides proper opportunities and presents means for satisfaction of our needs and desires. These needs may be biological, ethical or social. Culture has been defined as the process through which human beings satisfy their wants.
9. *Culture varies from society to society:* Every society has a culture of its own. Cultural elements, for example, customs, traditions, morals, ideas, values, ideologies, beliefs,

practices and institutions are different in each society. Culture also varies from time to time.

10. *Culture is super organic and ideational:* Culture is independent of physical and physiological properties and characteristics. The social meaning of a national flag is not just piece of coloured cloth. The flag represents the nation. Further every society considers its culture as an ideal. It is regarded as an end in itself.

Material and Non-material Aspects of Culture

Material culture consists of man-made objects such as tools, implements, automobiles, buildings, roads and all those devices by which nature is controlled. It is concerned with external, utilitarian and mechanical objects. It is referred as civilisation.

In non-material culture are included non-material objects like art, poetry and religion.

Cultural Lag

According to Ogburn, changes are quick to take place in the material culture. They in turn stimulate changes in the non-material culture. But the non-material culture may be slow to respond, giving rise to a gap or a lag between the material and non-material cultures. This lag is called the cultural lag.

Examples

1. The development in the field of industry requires a corresponding change in the system of education. The failure of education to cater to the needs of modern industrial development causes the "cultural lag".
2. Similarly, the forests of the country may be destroyed because the art of conservation does not keep pace with industrial or agricultural development.

Cultural Practices Influencing Health

Health beliefs and practices are part of every culture. Most ancient and some modern people believe that disease is due to wrath of some supernatural power. Even today, it is believed that venereal diseases and leprosy are punishments from God.

Scientific medicine conflicts with folk medicine, and their subcultures. Scientific health workers often fail because they do not realize that they are dealing with a subculture that must be sympathetically understood. Physicians and nurses must know the subculture with which they are dealing if they are to change the attitude of the patients towards hospital services.

The following cultural practices adversely affect family planning programmes:

a. Early marriage of the girl extents the reproductive period of the girl affecting her physical and mental maturity and health.
b. Preference for a male child prevents contraceptive practices for spacing, which is needed for regaining the health of the mother and provide her with free time for the first child.
c. Low status of women deprives her of basic nutritional food, shelter, clothing, education, freedom of speech, selection of mate and other important decision-making.
d. Taboos in discussing sexual problems openly results in increase in STDs and sex related health problems, further aggravating family welfare.

Following are cultural beliefs related to health:

1. Getting up early in the morning and taking bath.
2. Drinking Tulsi water every day for health.
3. Placing jasmine over the breast of postnatal woman will suppress the secretion of milk and consumption of garlic will produce more milk in lactating mother.
4. Circumcision of Muslim male child prevents urinary tract infection.
5. Eating papaya during the first trimester and last trimester will induce abortion and premature delivery.
6. Purdah system by Muslim women, causes Vitamin D deficiency.
7. Giving iron object during convulsion period will reduce intensity of fits.
8. Male child is preferred by Hindu parents for performing their last rites.

9. Periodic fasting will clean up the gastrointestinal tract. Weekly fasting by Hindu, during the month of Ramzan by Muslims and during lent by Christians.
10. Brahman and Vaisyas will not consume garlic, onions and non-vegetarian food.
11. Avoiding cold food (butter milk, curds, cucumber and guava during common cold).
12. Drum sticks will not be consumed by some sects.
13. Beet root consumption increases blood production in the body.
14. Alcoholism and drug abuse are indication of rich clan and complex society's culture.
15. Pregnant women eat mud/ash/chalk powder/lime powder (pica) as it enhances the normal development of foetus.

QUESTIONS

1. Mention any two specific beliefs in Indian culture which have adverse health effects.
2. What is community? Explain the elements of community.

29 Social Security

Social security has been defined as that security that society provides through appropriate organizations against certain risks to which its members are exposed. The risk covered in most countries by social security are sickness, invalidity, maternity, old age and death. Social security also includes social insurance and social assistance.

Social Security for Industrial Workers

The social security measures for industrial workers in India are contained in the following legislatures:

1. The Workmen's Compensation Act 1923
2. Employees State Insurance Act 1948
3. Central Maternity Benefit Act 1961
4. The Familly Pension Scheme 1971.

Social Welfare in India

Social welfare movement has gained ground in India like many other nations of the world. The planning commission was set up by the Government of India in March 1950 to prepare a plan for the most effective utilization of country's resources.

The department of social welfare created in 1964 and elevated to an independent ministry is responsible for general social welfare including nutrition programs for children and expectant mothers. It plans and coordinates the welfare services run by Government of India, the State Governments and National Voluntary agencies.

Welfare Programs

The various programs of social welfare services provided in India are classified under six heads.

1. Programs for the Welfare of Women
2. Programs for the Welfare of Children
3. Composite Programs for Women and Children.
4. Programs for the Maladjusted Groups
5. Programs for the Physically Handicapped Persons, e.g. blind, deaf, mentally challenged and orthopedically challenged.
6. Programs for the Welfare of Backward Classes.

Central Social Welfare Board

The Central Social Welfare board was set up in August 1953. It surveys the needs and requirements of Social Welfare Organizations in the country. It distributes funds to Voluntary Social Service Organizations for strengthening, improving and extending the existing activities in the field of Social welfare and for developing new programs and carrying out pilot projects.

Women Welfare

The department of Women and Child Development created in 1985 formulates and implements the policies and programs relating to women and child welfare.

Government of India Programs

The government of India has launched a number of program to eradicate the Poverty and Unemployment in India. The following are some of them:

1. Community Development Program launched on 2nd October 1951.
2. Integrated Rural Development Program (IRDP) launched during the 6th five year plan.
3. National Rural Employment Program (NREP).
4. Rural Landless Employment Guarantee Program

5. Tranining Program for Rural Youth for Self-employment
6. Jawahar Rogar Yojana (April 1989).
7. Jawahar Lal Nehru, National Urban Renewal Mission (Basic Services to the urban poor and integrated housing and slum development program).
8. Revised twenty point program.
9. Integrated Low Cost Sanitation (LCS) secheme with the goal of eradication of manual scavenging .
10. Rajiv Awas Yojana (RAY)
11. National Urban housing and Habitat policy with the goal of affordable housing for all.

Voluntary Organizations

Besides the Central and State Governments, more than 6000 Voluntary organization are also engaged in social welfare activities. Important voluntary organizations are:

1. The Indian Red Cross Society.
2. Bharat Sevak Samaj.
3. The Kasturba Memorial Fund.
4. Lions Club.
5. Ramakrishna Mission.
6. The Hind Kusht Nivaran Sangh.
7. Tuberculosis Association of India.
8. Indian Council for Child Welfare.
9. Family Planning Association of India.
10. All India Women's Conference.
11. The All India Blind Relief Society.

QUESTIONS

1. What is social security? Explain.
2 What is social planning? Explain.

30 Population Explosion

On May 11th, 2000 India's population reached one billion. According to UN projections, India's population will reach 1.52 billion by the year 2050 and will be the highest population in the world surpassing China. At present, India is the second most populous country, next to China, with only 2-4% of world land area, and supporting 16.87% of world population.

Causes of Rapid Growth of India's Population

1. High birth rate (22.8 per thousand at present) and decrease in death rate (9.1 per thousand at present). It was 43 per thousand in and 27 per thousand in 1951.
2. Early marriage (usually between 15-19 years).
3. Early puberty in Indian girls (12-13 years).
4. Child marriage, widow marriage, universal marriage.
5. Low level of literacy especially in rural areas.
6. Low standard of living. Where the standard of living is high, the birth rate tends to be low.
7. Lack of family planning.
8. Infant mortality.
9. Absence of social security.
10. Lack of recreational facilities.
11. Traditional customs and beliefs, e.g. desire for a male child, all women must marry.

Reasons for Falling Death Rate

1. Control over epidemics like smallpox, plague and cholera.
2. Progress in medical knowledge.

3. Extensive medical facilities for all.
4. Urbanization.

Life expectancy for Indian women is 67.5 years and 63.2 for men in 2012. The increase in life expectancy is due to better food supply and nutrition, healthier life styles and better hygiene.

Effect of Population Explosion on Economy

1. Not enough food and health services.
2. Not enough jobs, houses and schools.
3. Over-crowding in homes, hospitals, buses and trains.
4. Strain on public utility services such as electricity, water supply and sanitation.
5. Lower quality family life and health.
6. Lower living standards of the people.

Measures to Control the Rapidly Growing Population

India was the first country to adopt Family Planning Program in 1953. The average annual birth rate which was 42 per thousand population in 1951 has come down to 28.7 in 1993. The death rate also come down from 27/1000 to 9.3/1000 during the same period. Life expectancy in 2001 for males was 62.8 and for females 63.8. The current population pressures are seriously threatening the economic and social development of India and urgent and serious measures are required to control the population as follows:

1. Educational activities to create awareness and dessemination of specific information about family planning methods and the desirability of small family norms among the general masses.
2. Mass media has to be used extensively to propagate small family norm.
3. The raise in age at marriage has to be strictly enforced.
4. Strong disincentives for families with more than two children should be made available in public and private sectors.

5. Activities like film shows, exhibitions, mass meetings and group discussion about family planning should be organized more and more.
6. Highest priority should be given for Population Control Programs in our development plans.
7. Family Planning Program should be integrated with community health. People should understand that family planning implies planned family which serves as a basic pillar of planned economy.
8. The state should set up as many family planning centers as possible especially in rural areas.
9. Government have to inspire the professionals by giving awards and incentives for their excellent performance in the family welfare activities.
10. Religious leaders should be persuaded to advise small family norms in the larger interests of the community and the nation.
11. The recently introduced social welfare schemes like adult education, mahila mandals, cretches, bal wadies and loans to start self-employment by women, etc. have been helpful to bring about changes in peoples attitudes towards small family norms. More efforts in similar direction will go a long way for the success of family welfare and population control in India.

Literacy rate in India has gone up in 2012, to 74% from 65%. For males, it has risen by 7% from 75 to 82% and for females by 11% from 54 to 65% during the last on decade.

QUESTIONS

1. Explain social causes of population explosions. What are the consequences on health?
2. What are the health effects of child marriage?
3. Explain the causes of over population in India.

31 Health Economics

NATURAL RESOURCES

The word "economics" means house keeping. It deals with the human relationship in production, distribution, consumption and ownership of resources, goods and services. Economics and sociology are inseparable.

The process of economic development involves the growth of national output. To increase national output, it is essential to combine the natural resources, human resources and capital. Natural resources of a country determine the course of its development. India is very rich in natural resources and man power.

1. *Agriculture:* India's economy is heavily dependent on agriculture. It accounts for 46% of national income and employment for 52% of our population. The total agricultural area of India is 329 million hectares. About 47% of the available area is under cultivation. While India accounts for 17% of world population, it possesses only 2.4% of land resources of the world. The chances of increasing the cropped area are very limited and efforts are needed to intensify agriculture and increase productivity by double cropping and irrigation.
2. *Forest resources:* Forests have a modulating effect against floods and thereby protect the soil from erosion. Forests are a source of timber, bamboo, canes, kendu leaves, gums, resins, tanning material, rubber, dyes and honey. They provide raw materials to many important industries like furniture, matches, paper, rayon, tanning and construction. Total area under forests was 67 million hectares which was about 22% of the geographic area.

The tenth five year plan aimed at increasing the forest area to 25% of the geographical area.

3. *Fisheries:* India has a vast sea coast. The marine products feed the locals and earn foreign exchange. 1.8 million fishermen draw their livelihood from fisheries. Out of a total production of 28.5 lakh tons, 11 tons come from inland fisheries and 17.5 lakh tons from the sea. India produces only 9% of total supply of fish in Asia while Japan contributed 43% and China 18%.
4. *Water Resources:*

   Surface water: Total resources of surface water is estimated 168 million of which 33% is lost due to evaporation, 22% seeps into the soil and 45% flows to river basin and are available for irrigation.

   Underground water of the 36 million hectares of water seeping down the soil 20 lakhs are absorbed by the upper layers helping the growth of agriculture crops.

   Out of the total area of 140 million hectares under cultivation, only 45 million (i.e. only 33%) receives irrigation facilities from all the sources. Thus, there is a vast scope for expansion of irrigation.
5. *Power:* The commercial source of energy consists of coal, natural gas, hydroelectric power and nuclear fuel account for 45% of all energy or power consumption in India. Non-commercial sources of energy consists of firewood, charcoal, vegetable waste and dried cow dung and account for 35% of total power consumption. The balance 20% is made up of human effort and animal power. The power consumption in India is only 6% of Japan and 2.6% of the USA.
6. *Manpower:* The greatest natural resource of the country is its manpower. India's population stood at 1027 million in 2006. The people of India account for 17% of world population, while occupying only 2.4% of world's land area.

   Occupations: 52% of people in India are dependent on agriculture. The occupational status of India are as below:

Categories of workers	*% of total workers*
1. Cultivators	38.41
2. Agricultural labors	26.44

3. Livestock and forestry	1.90
4. Mining	0.62
5. House hold industry	2.42
6. Other than house hold industry	7.76
7. Constructions	1.94
8. Trade and commerce	7.46
9. Transport and communication	2.81
10. Other workers	10.23

Per Capita Income

Per capita income refers to the average income per head in a country. It is obtained by dividing the national income by the total population. As population increases the national income also increases substantially, but the per capita income may not increase. It may even fall if the growth of population is too high. It is because the national income gets distributed among the large population. Per capita income of India is very low, as India has low national income but the second largest population in the world. The national for capita monthly income 2011–12 was ₹ 5130. The 11th five year plan aims at doubling the per capita income.

QUESTION

1. Write briefly about India's natural resources and how they help the economic development of our country. What is per capita income?

32 Budgeting for a Family

FAMILY BUDGET

Family budget is an estimate of family income from various sources and an estimate of distribution of family expenditure on various items for a specified period of time, for example, a month or a year depending upon the size of family income and expenditure. A family with a large income and various types of expenditure of bigger size will have a budget for the shorter period as compared to a family with less income and fewer items of expenditure.

One should cut his coat according to his cloth. According to the availability of income, the house wife should prepare her budget. The family budget should be discussed and planned by the whole family, so that each member of the family understands his individual responsibility in making the budget a success.

Principle of planning a budget: Budget for a month or year depends on:

1. The total amount of income
2. Different sources of the income
3. Size of the family
4. Status of family
5. Provision for the future.

Steps in preparing a budget:

1. Record income from all the sources.
2. List all fixed expenditure and estimated anticipated expenses.
3. Study the present spending habits of the family and the areas, if any, where the expenditure can be curtailed.
4. Study the unusual anticipated expenditure to determine whether the satisfaction reached would justify the expenditure.

5. Find out the best mode of investing at least 15% of the family income on long-term deposits for rainy days, i.e. for unforeseen future expenditure.

Items of Expenditure

The main items of expenditure in the family are food, house rent, electricity charges, and school fees of children. Each family should try to make the best use of the estimated income. The family spends the largest portion of its income on food (Table 32.1).

Health of the family is the most important goal of the family budget. All the money spent on medicines, medical check-up, fees of doctors, dentists, hospital charges, special diet for the sick members of the family, tonics recommended by the doctors, various types of soaps, shampoos and oils used by the family members for their personal care come as expenditure under health. If any member has been advised to stay at a health resort for some time or special diet, such expenditure also will be considered as an expenditure on health.

Table 32.1: Percent of distribution of income

Items of expenditure	For a family with monthly income above ₹ 6,000/- (in %)
Food	33
House	18
Clothing	12
Education	9
Health	7
Recreation	6
Miscellaneous	6
Savings	15

Advantages of Making a Family Budget

1. Budgeting helps the family to spend the money carefully and keep the expenditure within its means.
2. Budget is a good guide for family expenditure.
3. It brings balance between current and future expenses of the family.

4. It prevents the family from extravagant expenditure and fall into debt trap.
5. It ensures balanced spending and ensures expenditure on priority items.
6. Members of the family realise their individual responsibilities in sharing their income.
7. It relieves the earning family members from meeting the demands and expectation from time to time.
8. Members of the family learns the value and virtue of cooperation.
9. The family budget provides a record of the family expenditure of that period for future references.
10. The biggest advantage of the family budget is that it enables the family to live within their means and be healthier and happier.

QUESTION

1. Explain the method of preparing a planned budget for the family.

Board Question Papers

Armed Forces Medical Services Examining Board First Year GNM Examination for Probationer Nurses and Nursing Assistants: August 2007

Paper II: Behavioural Sciences

Time: 3 Hours Max. Marks: 75

Instructions:

1. Answer to Part—I and Part II to be written in separate answer books.
2. Figures to the right indicate full marks.
3. All questions are compulsory.
4. Draw neat diagrams where necessary.

Part-I: Psychology

Marks

1. a. i. Define learning. 1
   ii. Describe factors of effective learning. 4
   iii. Discuss the laws of effective learning with suitable illustrations involving patients. 10

OR

   b. i. Define Psychology. 1
   ii. Describe the branches of psychology. 4
   iii. How psychology will help the student nurse in her development as a care giver. 10

2. Write short answers for any **FIVE**: 3×5=15
   a. How can you have control over your emotions?
   b. Describe in brief the personality traits expected in a nurse.
   c. What are the attitudes needed to become a seccessful and efficient nurse?

d. Discuss in brief the James' Maxims of habit formation.
e. Describe the stages involved in problem solving.
f. Analyse the factors that control and direct goal directed attention.

3. Fill in the blanks: 1×5=5
   a. An attitude of hatred towards a certain community is a .... attitude.
   b. Day dreaming is dreaming during ....
   c. In .... , the thought processes are allowed greater freedom of action.
   d. Mental age concept is first brought by ....
   e. .... works on pleasure principle.

4. Match column 'B' with column 'A': 1×5=5

A	B	
a. Psychoanalytic theory	i. Pyknic type	( )
b. Learning by conditioning	ii. Freud	( )
c. Kretschmer	iii. Rationalisation	( )
d. Sour-Grapes	iv. Displacement	( )
e. Projection	v. Pavlov	( )

Part-II: Sociology

1. a. Define family. 2
   b. Functions of a family. 5
   c. Merits and demerits of joint family. 8

2. Write short note on any **THREE**: 5×3=15
   a. Social disorganization.
   b. Primary group.
   c. Difference between caste and class.
   d. Values and Mores.
   e. Social security.

3. Tick (✓) the right answer: 1×5=15
   a. Theory of cultural lag is propounded by:
      i. Maciver
      ii. Ogburn

   iii. Gillin-Gillin
   iv. Fairchild

b. Origin of society was due to:
   i. Force
   ii. God's will
   iii. Evolution
   iv. Culture

c. Which of the following is an informal method of social control:
   i. Belief
   ii. Law
   iii. Coercion
   iv. Education

d. Social process takes place when there is:
   i. Integration
   ii. Competition
   iii. Assimilation
   iv. None of the above

e. Punishment for demanding dowry is:
   i. Imprisonment extending 6 months
   ii. Penalty exceeding ₹ 5,000.

Karnataka State Diploma in Nursing Examining Board
February 2007 (New Syllabus)
1st Year—Paper-II
Behavioural Science—Psychology and Sociology

Time: 3 Hours | Max. Marks: 75
Psychology: 50
Sociology: 25

Section-I (38 Marks)

Psychology

I. Give the meaning of the following terms: 1×5=5
   a. Motivation.
   b. Mental health.
   c. Skills.
   d. Memory.
   e. Observation or Aptitude.

II. Fill in the blanks with suitable word or words: 1×5=5
   a. Father of analytical psychology is ....
   b. .... is an example of frustration
   c. .... is an example of anti-social behaviour
   d. Intelligence quotient was first measured by ....
   e. Science of population is known as ....

III. Write short notes on the following: 5×3=15
   a. Effects of emotional reactions.
   b. Steps involved in learning process.
   c. Conflicts.

IV. a. List adjustment mechanisms. 2+5=7
   b. Briefly state two examples of mental mechanisms.

V. a. Define attention. 2+4=6
   b. Write briefly the factors affecting attention.

OR

   a. Define perception. 2+4=6
   b. Explain briefly the errors of perception.

Section–II (37 Marks)

Sociology

VI. Give the meaning of the following: 1×5=5

a. Social psychology.
b. Joint family.
c. Marriage.
d. Dowry.
e. Observation.

VII. Write short notes on any **THREE** of the following: 5×3=15

a. Resources of the country.
b. Alcoholism.
c. Basic needs of family.
d. Importance of sociology.
e. Rights and responsibilities of a citizen.

VIII. a. Define culture. 2+4+4=10
b. List the elements of culture.
c. Write its characteristics.

IX. a. Define community. 2+5=7
b. List the characteristics of community.

OR

a. Define social control. 2+2+3=7
b. List the purpose of social control.
c. Write the characteristics of social control.

Karnataka State Diploma in Nursing Examination Board
August 2007 GNM Examination (New Syllabus)
1st Year—Paper-II
Psychology and Sociology

Max. Marks:75
Time: 3 Hours Psychology: 50
Sociology: 25

Section–I (38 Marks)

I. Give the meaning of the following: 1×4=4
a. Child psychology.
b. Maladjustment.
c. Attitude.
d. Frustration.

II. State whether the following statements are True or False: 1×4=4
a. Moods affect our normal behaviour.
b. IQ of moron is 51 to 71%.
c. Lacking concentration is not an attention disorder.
d. Ivan Pavlov is known for his work in psychoanalysis.

III. Write short notes on any **THREE** the following: 5×3=15
a. Conflicts.
b. Intelligence tests.
c. Importance of psychology in nursing profession.
d. Dynamics of human behaviour.

IV. a. What is an emotion? 2+6+6=14
b. Discuss three examples of emotion.
c. How to control emotions?

V. a. What is learning? 2+5+6=13
b. State laws of learning.
c. Enumerate factors promoting effective learning.

Section–II (37 Marks)

VI. Give the meaning of the following: 1×4=4

a. Sociology.
b. Deliquency.
c. Tradition.
d. Social change.

VII. State whether the statements are True or False: 1×3=3

a. Culture is not inherited.
b. Every group is dependent upon other group.
c. Community has no locality limitation.

VIII. Write short notes on any **TWO** of the following: 3×2=6

a. Nature of family.
b. Rights and responsibilities of individuals in a democratic society.
c. Group morale.

IX. a. Define Society. 1+2+3=6

b. Describe elements of society.
c. Explain briefly its characteristics.

X. a. List social problems. 3+3=6

b. Explain briefly any one social problem.

Karnataka State Diploma in Nursing Examination Board
1st Year Behavioural Science—Psychology and Sociology (Paper-II) February 2008

Max. Marks: 75
Time: 3 Hours Psychology: 50
Sociology: 25

Section–I (50 Marks)

Psychology

I. Give the meaning of the following terms: 1×5=5
   a. Conflict.
   b. Introspection.
   c. Intelligence.
   d. Behaviour.
   e. Skills.

II. State whether the following are True or False: 1×5=5
   a. After menopause a woman experiences chage in her pattern of life.
   b. In old age physical capacity increases.
   c. Adler introduced to measure general intelligence.
   d. Concentration is difficult when one is having a state of fatigue.
   e. In interaction, mental functions and physical conditions are affected.

III. Write short notes on any **TWO** the following: 3×2=6
   a. Attitudes.
   b. Problem solving techniques.
   c. Advantages and disadvantages of habits.

IV. a. Define psychology. 2+3+3=8
   b. State different branches of psychology.
   c. Write briefly about each of them.

V. a. Define motive. 2+2+4=8
   b. Elaborate the classification of motives.
   c. Briefly describe any two motives.

VI. a. Define thinking. 2+2+2=8
b. Describe briefly free thinking.
c. Describe the types of thinking.

Section–II (25 Marks)

Sociology

VII. Fill in the blanks: 1×4=4
a. .... is the father of sociology.
b. .... and .... are the branches of social sciences.
c. Head of the family in matriarchal family is the ....
d. .... is required for socialization of individuals.

VIII. State whether the following are True or False: 1×4=4
a. Language is the main media of culture.
b. Polygamy is not practiced amongst various religions.
c. Changes in environment, change the social behaviour of man.
d. Population explosion hinders the progress of the nation as a whole.

IX. Write short notes on any **FOUR** of the following:

3×4=12
a. Economic aspects of community and its effects on health and illness.
b. Rural and urban society.
c. Characteristics of marriage.
d. Family life education.
e. Resources of the country.

X. a. Define Group. 2+5+2=9
b. Briefly explain types of groups.
c. Give the characteristics of groups.

XI. a. List social changes in community. 4+4=8
b. Write briefly about the ways and means of social control.

Karnataka State Diploma in Nursing Examination Board August 2008 GNM Examination (New Syllabus) 1st Year—Paper-II Behavioural Science—Psychology and Sociology

Time: 3 Hours | Max. Marks: 75
Psychology: 50
Sociology: 25

Section-I —Psychology

I. Give the meaning of the following: 1×5=5
  a. Hallucination.
  b. Attention.
  c. Psychology.
  d. Mental health.
  e. Defence Mechanism.

II. Fill in the blanks with suitable answer: 1×5=5
  a. .... is the physiological motive.
  b. .... are drugs which alter consciousness.
  c. False perception is ....
  d. Conflicts are of .... forms.
  e. An inner force which drives an individual to certain action is known as ....

III. State whether the following statement are True or False: 1×5=5
  a. Habits are the time and energy saving techniques.
  b. Paresthesia is false sensation.
  c. Motivation is a negative feeling.
  d. Depth perception is also known as third dimension.
  e. Thinking, reasoning promotes effective learning.

IV. Write short notes on any **THREE** of the following: 5×3=15
  a. Intelligence and its tests.
  b. Counselling and its characteristics.

c. Laws of effective learning.
d. Psychosis and its types.

V. a. What is drug abuse and drug addict? 2+3+5=10
b. Mention its causes.
c. Explain the preventive measures.

VI. a. What is Personality? 2+3+5=10
b. Mention the types of personality.
c. Explain the factors influencing personality.

Section–II—Sociology

VII. Write short notes on any **TWO** of the following: 4×2=8

a. Social group.
b. Family and its types.
c. Marriage.

VIII. a. What is population explosion? 2+5=7
b. Write its effect on the society.

IX. a. Enumerate the social problems of society. 2+8=10
b. Explain in detail about dowry system, alcoholism and deliquency.

Karnataka State Diploma in Nursing Examination Board, Bengaluru
February 2009 GNM Examination
1st Year—Paper
Behavioural Science—Psychology and Sociology

Time: 3 Hours Max. Marks: 75

Section-I

I. Give the meaning of the following: 1×4=4
   a. IQ.
   b. Emotion.
   c. Illusion.
   d. Observation.

II. State whether the following are True or False: 1×4=4
   a. Habits are learned behaviour.
   b. Philosphy is the part of psychology.
   c. Mental, physical and emotional function are closely related.
   d. The word psychology is derived from Latin word "Psyche" and "Logos".

III. Write short notes on any **TWO** of the following: 5×2=10
   a. Scope of psychology.
   b. Dynamics of behaviour.
   c. Motives.

IV. a. Define intelligence. 1+4+5=10
   b. Explain the branches of psychology.
   c. Write the uses of psychology in nursing.

V. a. Define intelligence. 2+3+5=10
   b. Write the nature of intelligence.
   c. Explain bell-shapped curve distribution of intelligence.

Section–II

VI. Define the following: 1×3=3

a. Sociology.
b. Personality.
c. Culture.

VII. Fill in the blanks with suitable words: 1×4=4

a. ....is called father of sociology.
b. Marriage is .... between man and woman.
c. The study of sociology helps the nurse to identify.........
d. The word personality is derived from ....word persona.

VIII. Write short notes on any **TWO** of the following: 5 × 2 = 10

a. Family.
b. Folk ways.
c. Delinquency.

IX. a. Define urban community. 2+4+4=10

b. Write the characteristics of urban community.
c. Mention the social problems in the urban community.

X. a. Explain Carl Jung's classification of personality. 3+7=10

b. Write the characteristic features of each type of this classification.

Karnataka State Diploma in Nursing Examination Board
August 2009 GNM Examination (New Syllabus)
1st Year—Paper-II
Psychology and Sociology

Time: 3 Hours Max. Marks: 75

Section–I

I. Fill up the blanks:
  a. Intelligence quotent was first measured by .... and..........
  b. False perception with presence of object is called........
  c. An attitude of respect towards elders is a .... attitude.
  d. ....is known as father of mental health.

II. State whether the following statements are True or False:
  a. False unshakable belief is known as delusion.
  b. Response to the stimulus is known as behaviour.
  c. Sigmund Freud is known for classical conditioning.
  d. IQ of normal individual is 51 to 71.

III. Write short notes on any two of the following: 5×2=10
  a. Habits.
  b. Types of learning.
  c. Development of intelligent behaviour.

IV. a. Define psychology. 2+3+5=10
  b. Mention the scope of psychology.
  c. How does the knowledge of psychology is helpful in nursing?

V. a. Define motives. 2+3+5=10
  b. How are they classified?
  c. What is the importance of motives in patient care?

Section-II

VI. Fill up the blanks with suitable answers: 1×3=3

a. .... is the father of sociology.

b. ....consists of husband, wife and their offsprings.

c. ....and .... are responsible for national economy.

VII. State whether the following statements are True or False: 1×4=4

a. Personality is physical attraction of an individual.

b. Culture influences behaviour and health programs of the population.

c. Community has definite geographical locality.

d. Culture is inherited.

VIII. Write short notes on any **TWO**: 4×2=8

a. Functions of the family.

b. Rights and responsibilities of an individual in a democratic society.

c. Difference between rural and urban society.

IX. a. Enumerate the social problems of society. 4+6=10

b. Explain any two of the problems.

X. a. Define personality. 2+4+6=12

b. Mention the types of personality.

c. Explain the factors influencing the personality.

Karnataka State Diploma in Nursing Examination Board, Bengaluru February 2010 GNM Examination 1st Year—Paper-II Psychology and Sociology

Time: 3 Hours | Max. Marks: 75

Section–I

I. Fill up the blanks: 1×4=4

a. Intelligence quotent was first measured by .... and ....

b. False perception with presence of object is called........

c. An Attitude of respect towards elders is a .... attitude.

d. ....is known as Father of mental health.

II. State whether the following statements are True or False:

1×4=4

a. False unshakable belief is known as delusion.

b. Response to the stimulus is known as behaviour.

c. Sigmund Freud is known for classical conditioning.

d. IQ of normal individual is 51 to 71.

III. Write short notes on any **TWO** of the following: 5×2=10

a. Habits.

b. Types of learning.

c. Development of intelligent behaviour.

IV. a. Define psychology. 2+3+5=10

b. Mention the scope of psychology.

c. How does the knowledge of psychology is helpful in nursing.

V. a. Define motives. 2+3+5=10

b. How are they classified?

c. What is the importance of motives in patient care?

Section–II

VI. Fill up the blanks with suitable answers: 1×3=3

a........................... is the father of sociology.

b. ....consists of husband, wife and their offsprings.

c. ....and .... are responsible for national economy.

VII. State whether the following statements are True or False: 1×4=4

a. Personality is physical attraction of an individual.

b. Culture influences behaviour and health programs of the population.

c. Community has definite geographical locality.

d. Culture is inherited.

VIII. Write short notes on any **TWO**: 4×2=8

a. Functions of the family.

b. Rights and responsibilities of an individual in a democratic society.

c. Difference between rural and urban society.

IX. a. Enumerate the social problems of society. 4+6=10

b. Explain any two of the problems.

X. a. Define personality. 2+4+6=12

b. Mention the types of personality.

c. Explain the factors influencing the personality.

Karnataka State Diploma in Nursing Examination Board August 2010 GNM Examination 1st Year—Paper-II Psychology and Sociology

Time: 3 Hours | Max. Marks:75

Section-I

I. Fill up the blanks: 1×5=5

a. The word psychology is derived from two Greek words .... and ....

b. ....is loss of memory.

c. ....is an inaccurate perception.

d. Father of psychology is ....

II. State whether the following statements are True or False: 1×4=4

a. Defence mechanisms are known as mental mechanisms.

b. Habit is recurring acquired mode of behaviour.

c. Formula used to measure IQ is:

$$IQ = \frac{CA}{MA} \times 100$$

d. Hyperthesia means loss of response to stimuli.

III. Write short notes on any **THREE** of the following: 5×3=15

a. Factors that control and direct attention.

b. Sources and nature of frustration.

c. Factors that determine our attitude.

d. Development of intellegent behaviour.

IV. a. Define emotions and feelings. 1+2+4=7

b. How are emotions classified and expressed?

c. Write the effect of emotional reactions on health.

V. a. What is adjustment? 2+2+4=8

b. Explain the common defense mechanism.

c. Write the importance of adjustment.

Section-II

VI. Fill up the blanks with suitable answers: 1×3=3

a. One who shows deviation from normal behaviour is..........

b. Study of population is called as ....

c. Average income per person in a year is called as .... income.

VII. State whether the following statements are True or False: 1×4=4

a. Polygamy is practiced among all religions.

b. Hippocrates is the father of medicine.

c. Population explosion hinders the progress of that nation as whole.

d. In monogamy one man marries only on woman.

VIII. Write short notes on any **TWO** of the following: 5×2=10

a. Explain the types of family and basic needs of family.

b. Social changes.

c. Culture and the characteristics of culture.

IX. a. Define personality. 2+3+5=10

b. Write the components of personality.

c. Explain the factors influencing personality.

X. a. Define society. 2+3+5=10

b. Write the elements.

c. Describe the rights and responsibilities of an individual in a democratic society.

Karnataka State Diploma in Nursing Examination Board
February 2011 GNM Examination
1st Year—Paper-II
Psychology and Sociology

Time: 3 Hours Max. Marks: 75

Section–I

I. Give the meaning of the following: 1×5=5

a. Psychology.
b. Memory.
c. Frustration.
d. Forgetting.

II. Fill in the blanks: 1×6=6

a. Emotions are classified in to .... and ....
b. Attitudes accompanied by strong feelings are called ....
c. Three types of habits are......................, ... and ....

III. Write short notes on any **THREE** of the following: 5×3=15

a. Factors that promote effective learning.
b. Factors affecting development of personality.
c. Importance of psychology in nursing profession.
d. Conflicts.

IV. a. What is mental mechanism? 2+4=6
b. Explain any three mechnisms with examples.

V. a. Define Hallucination. 1+5=6
b. Write the various types of hallucination with examples.

Section–II

VI. Choose the correct answer: 1×3=3

a. The term embryo means
i. From 3 months to birth.

   ii. Conception to 12 weeks of intrauterine life.
   iii. From birth to 1 month.

b. The word family has been taken from
   i. Latin
   ii. Roman
   iii. Greek.

c. One woman marries many men and lives with them as their wife.
   i. Polygamy
   ii. Polyandry
   iii. Endogamy.

VII. Fill in the blanks: $1 \times 5 = 5$

a. One who shows deviation from normal behavior is called ....

b. Demography is the scientific study of............................

c. Prostitution is considered as one of the .... profession.

d. Two types of economical aspects of individuals are .... and ....

VIII. Write short notes on any **THREE** of the following: 5×3=15

a. Fundamental rights and responsibilities of an individual in a democratic society.

b. Factors influencing the growth and development.

c. Difference between rural and urban society.

d. Unmarried mothers.

IX. a. Define community. 2+6=8

b. Write the characteristics and types of community.

X. a. Define family. 1+5=6

b. Write the types of family and its functions.

Karnataka State Diploma in Nursing Examination Board
August 2011 GNM Examination
1st Year—Paper-II
Behaviour Sciences—Psychology and Sociology

Time: 3 Hours Max. Marks: 75

Section-I

I. Give the meaning of the following: 1×4=4
   a. Legal psychology.
   b. Skills.
   c. Habits.
   d. Introspection.

II. Fill in the blanks: 1×4=4
   a. Forgetfulness is due to lack of ....
   b. Unattainable goals can be important sources of ....
   c. Illusions are ....
   d. .... is a loss of memory.

III. Write short notes on any **THREE** of the following: 5×3=15
   a. Branches of psychology.
   b. Perception.
   c. Conflicts.
   d. Development of intelligent behaviours.

IV. a. Define Emotion. 1+3+4=8
   b. List the characteristics of an emotion.
   c. Explain the role of a nurse in control of emotion.

V. a. Define learning. 1+2+4=7
   b. Mention the types of learning.
   c. Explain the factors influencing learning.

Section-II

VI. Choose the correct answer and write: 1×3=3
   a. .... is widely spread in tribal society.
      i. Illiteracy

ii. Literacy
iii. Ignorance

b. Prostitution is a social problem and it is due to:
i. Urge
ii. Rituals
iii. Poverty

c. Urban community means an area with:
i. High population density
ii. Low population density
iii. Both

VII. State whether the following statements are True or False: 1×4=4

a. Web of social relations is called society.
b. Primary group is a group where there is face to face contact and reciprocal communication.
c. HIV can be transmitted by hugging, shaking hands and sharing home with an infected person.
d. Premarriage counselling is necessary to build a healthy marriage and to reduce the number of divorces.

VIII. Write short notes on any **TWO** of the following: 5×2=10

a. Importance of sociology in nursing.
b. Alcoholism.
c. Budgeting for a family.

IX. a. Define social control. 2+3+5=10

b. List the purposes of social control.
c. Briefly explain the means of social control.

OR

a. Define culture.
b. List the functions of culture.
c. Write the characteristics of culture.

X. a. Define Personality. 2+2+6=10

b. List the types of personality.
c. Explain the factors affecting development of personality.

Karnataka State Diploma in Nursing Examination Board
February 2012 GNM Examination
1st Year—Paper-II
Behaviour Sciences—Psychology and Sociology

Time: 3 Hours Max. Marks: 75

Section—I

I. Give the meaning of the following: 1×4=4
   a. Mental health.
   b. Behaviour.
   c. Emotion.
   d. Frustration.

II. Fill in the blanks: 1×4=4
   a. IQ of a imbecile is ....
   b. Habits are a form of our .... behaviour.
   c. Illusions are .... perceptions.
   d. The word "Loci" means................................

III. Write short notes on any **TWO** of the following: 5×2=10
   a. Memory.
   b. Attitude.
   c. Types of learning.

IV. a. Define psychology. 2+2+6=10
   b. List out the branches of psychology.
   c. Explain in detail the importance of psychology in nursing.

V. a. Define conflicts. 2+3+5=10
   b. Enumerate the types of conflicts.
   c. Explain the measures to overcome frustration and conflicts.

Section—II

VI. Fill in the blanks: 1×3=3
   a. Dowry Prohibition Act is passed on ....
   b. A man who marries two women is called................

c. Scientific study of human population is called.....................

VII. State whether the following statements are True or False: 1×4=4

a. In our India we have more than 300 castes and sub castes.
b. Culture is derived from Greek word.
c. GNP means gross national product.
d. The other name for nuclear family is conjugal family.

VIII. Write short notes on any **TWO** of the following: 4×2=8

a. Social change.
b. Prostitution.
c. Types of family.

IX. a. Define community. 2+4+4=10
b. Mention the characteristics of community.
c. Explain the differences between rural community and urban community.

X. a. Define personality. 1+5+6=12
b. List the factors affecting development of personality.
c. Explain Carl Jung classification of personality.

Karnataka State Diploma in Nursing Examination Board
August 2012 GNM Examination
1st Year—Paper-II
Behaviour Sciences—Psychology and Sociology

Time: 3 hours Max. Marks: 75

SECTION—I

I. Choose the correct answer and write: 1×4=4

a. Initially psychology was considered as science
   i. Mild.
   ii. Soul.
   iii. Brain.

b. Emotion word was derived from:
   i. Greek.
   ii. Latin.
   iii. France.

c. Learning is growth through:
   i. Learning.
   ii. Experience.
   iii. Behaviour.

d. Formula for IQ:
   i. $\frac{MA}{CA} \times 100$
   ii. $\frac{MA}{CA} \times 10$
   iii. $\frac{CA}{MA} \times 100$

II. Fill in the blanks: 1×4=4

a. Genetic psychology is also called as..................
b. Excessive response to stimuli is known as.....................
c. In unconscious mind the conflicts are ....
d. Thinking is a .... mental activity.

III. Write short notes on any **THREE** of the following: 5×3=15

a. Adjustment mechanisms.
b. Advantages and limitations of intelligence tests.
c. Forgetfulness.
d. Factors affecting perception.

IV. a. Define memory. 1+3+4=8
b. Enumerate the types of memory.
c. Explain the techniques to improve memory.

V. a. Define motivation. 1+3+3=7
b. Write the types of motives.
c. Briefly explain about psychosocial motives.

Section-II

VI. Differentiate between the following: 2×4=8

a. Nuclear family	and	Joint family
b. Growth	and	Development
c. Caste	and	Class
d. Extrovert	and	Introvert

VII. Write short notes on any **THREE** of the following: 4×3=12
a. Women abuse.
b. Functions of family.
c. Population control.
d. The rights and responsibilities of the individual in a democratic country.

VIII. a. Define economy. 1+3+5=9
b. List the essential elements of family budgeting.
c. What are the advantages of planning budget for a family?

IX. a. Differentiate between pyknic and asthenic personality.

2+6=8

b. Mention the commonly used techniques for assessing personality.

Karnataka State Diploma in Nursing Examination Board
June 2013 GNM Supplementary Examination
1st Year—Paper-II
Behaviour Sciences—Psychology and Sociology

Time: 3 Hours Max. Marks: 75

Section-I

I. Give the meaning of the following: 1×4=4
   a. Behaviour.
   b. Memory.
   c. Mental health.
   d. Motivation.

II. Fill in the blanks: 1×4=4
   a. .... is also known as daydreaming.
   b. .... is a mistaken perception.
   c. ....means soul and mind.
   d. An attitude of respect towards the elders is ....

III. Write short notes on any **THREE** of the following: 5×3=15
   a. Factors promoting effective learning.
   b. Errors in perception.
   c. Development of intelligent behaviour.
   d. Advantage and disadvantage of habit formation.

IV. a. What is emotion? 1+3+4=8
   b. How it differs from feeling?
   c. Explain the internal changes in emotional reactions.

V. a. What is psychology? 2+5=7
   b. Explain the scope of psychology.

Section-II

VI. Choose the correct answer and write: 1×3=3
   a. The great philosopher remarked that man is a social animal
      i. Aristotle.

   ii. Gillins and Gillins.
   iii. John Cuber.
b. Large number of people gathered in one place is called
   i. Crowd.
   ii. Pubic.
   iii. Gathering.
c. The Special Marriage Act was passed by the Government of India in the year
   i. 1954.
   ii. 1961.
   iii. 1970.

VII. State whether the following statements are True or False: 1×4=4
   a. Polygamy is practiced in all religions.
   b. Primary group is small in size.
   c. Rural community is heterogenous.
   d. Socialization is a learning process.

VIII. Write short notes on any **TWO** of the following: 5×2=10
   a. Uses of sociology in nursing profession.
   b. Population explosion.
   c. Budgeting for the family.

IX. a. Define society. 2+3+5=10
   b. Write the characteristics of society.
   c. Explain any three social problems faced in the society.

OR

   a. Define family.
   b. Mention the types and write the characteristics.
   c. Explain the family life education.

X. a. Define personality development. 2+3+5=10
   b. Write the classification of any one type (Sheldon classification OR Sigmund Freud's classification).
   c. Explain the factors affecting development of personality.

INDEX

Page numbers followed by *f* refer to figure and *t* refer to table